Fegan's Compression Sclerotherapy for Varicose Veins

Springer
London
Berlin
Heidelberg
New York
Hong Kong
Milan
Paris
Tokyo

Shukri K. Shami and Timothy R. Cheatle (Eds)

Fegan's Compression Sclerotherapy for Varicose Veins

With 30 Figures
including 26 colour plates

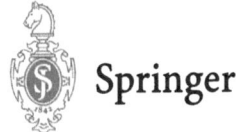 Springer

Shukri K. Shami, MB BS, FRCS(Ed), MS
Consultant Vascular Surgeon, Department of Surgery, Oldchurch Hospital,
Romford, Essex, UK

Timothy R. Cheatle, MS FRCS(I)
Consultant Vascular Surgeon, Department of Surgery, Oldchurch Hospital,
Romford, Essex, UK

Cover illustration: Portrait of Professor George Fegan by Yago Casado

British Library Cataloguing in Publication Data
Fegan's compression sclerotherapy for varicose veins.
  1. Injections, Sclerosing 2. Varicose veins – Treatment
  I. Shami, Shukri K., 1952– II. Cheatle, Timothy R. III. Fegan,
  George. Varicose veins IV. Compression sclerotherapy for
  varicose veins
  616.1′43

ISBN 978-1-4471-3475-6   ISBN 978-1-4471-3473-2 (eBook)
DOI 10.1007/978-1-4471-3473-2

Library of Congress Cataloging-in-Publication Data
A catalog record for this book is available from the Library of Congress

a member of BertelsmannSpringer Science+Business Media GmbH
www.springer.co.uk

Typeset by EXPO Holdings, Malaysia

Foreword

It may be surprising that a French vascular surgeon has been asked to write the foreword for an English book devoted to sclerotherapy. Nevertheless I have been delighted to fulfill this task.

As the authors state, this book is not a textbook but it is a "goldmine" of knowledge covering many aspects of phlebology.

The chapters on anatomy, histology and applied physiology give outstanding information usually not found in books devoted to phlebology. The sections on venous investigations and compression treatment are both clearly explained. The promoter of compression sclerotherapy, George Fegan, details both the technique and indications of his own treatment method; the literature review on sclerotherapy by TR. Cheatle is exhaustive and perfectly analysed. He stresses the fact that there have been no prospective randomized trials assessing the treatment results of modern varicose vein surgery and sclerotherapy.

I am convinced that all physicians interested in chronic venous disorders will enjoy the revised edition of "Compression Sclerotherapy for Varicose Veins" amongst other thoughtful analyses of venous disease.

Michel Perrin MD
Vascular Surgeon & Founding President of European Venous Forum
Chassieu
France

Preface

Nearly 40 years have passed since the first edition of this text appeared. In preparing this new edition, we have included new chapters on subjects in which significant increases in our knowledge have been made – physiology, the effects of compression on the microcirculation, and techniques of investigation. Professor George Fegan's original description of his method of performing sclerotherapy remains largely unchanged.

The book is not a textbook; it is centred on one man's description of the technique he developed. George Fegan is an enthusiast, and it has been a great privilege to work with him in the preparation of this edition. Sclerotherapy has been the subject of both uncritical adulation and unfair denigration over the past half-century. Slowly – more slowly than George Fegan would have wished – it is finding its place as an effective weapon in the phlebologist's armamentarium, and its indications are becoming clearer.

We hope this book will be of interest to all those involved in the care of patients with venous disease, and that it will stimulate further appraisal of Fegan's technique of sclerotherapy.

Thanks are due to Mr Robert Gardiner for facilitating this second edition, Dr John Farrah for the duplex images in Chapter 4, Dr Mary Henry for allowing us to use her photographs in Chapter 7, and Dr N. Bhardraj for help in obtaining references for the literature review.

Shukri Shami
Timothy Cheatle

Contents

Contents

Contributors

A Abu-Own PhD, FRCS
Consultant Vascular Surgeon
Ipswich Hospital NHS Trust
Ipswich, Suffolk
UK

Timothy R Cheatle MCh, FRCS(I)
Consultant Vascular Surgeon
Department of Surgery
Oldchurch Hospital
Romford, Essex
UK

George Fegan, MCh, FRCSI
Emeritus Professor of Surgery, Trinity College Dublin
Retired Consultant Surgeon, Sir Patrick Dun's Hospital, Rotunda Hospital
and Drogheda Cottage Hospital
Dublin
Ireland

Michel Perrin
Founding president, European Venous Forum
Unite de pathologie vasculaire Jean Kunlin
Clinique du grand large
Lyon
France

Colin A Rogers FRCS
Consultant Vascular Surgeon
Queen's Hospital
Burton on Trent, Staffordshire
UK

I Saeed FRCPath, FFPath
Consultant Histopathologist
Harold Wood Hospital
Romford, Essex
UK

Sanjeev Sarin MS, FRCS
Consultant Vascular Surgeon
Watford General Hospital
Watford, Hertfordshire
UK

Shukri K Shami MB, BS, FRCS(Ed), MS
Consultant Vascular Surgeon
Department of Surgery
Oldchurch Hospital
Romford, Essex
UK

Introduction

In order to understand the cause of varicose veins, one must understand the different factors that give rise to symmetrical hypertrophic dilation and to asymmetrical atrophic dilation. One factor is due to changes in pressure and the other is due to changes in flow. Symmetrical hypertrophic dilation produces valvular incompetence due to the dilation of the valve ring; it is reversible. The incompetence due to thrombosis and recanalisation is not reversible. The reversible valvular incompetence follows upward dilation and results from the irreversible valvular incompetence of a valve in a perforating vein. The two forms of valvular incompetence are due to two different causes.

Retrograde turbulent flow produces its effect in medium-sized, badly supported, superficial veins; the vibration of the turbulence produces muscle atrophy in the vessel wall, followed by stretching of the collagen fibres and the development of a bulge in the vein wall. Abnormal flow produces change in the poorly supported superficial veins. This is demonstrated most clearly in the development of a saphena varix, which can disappear following reduction in diameter and restoration of valvular competence.

Symmetrical upward dilation is due to an increase in the diameter of the vein as a result of an increase in the workload; it produces reversible valvular incompetence. Thrombosis and recanalisation produce irreversible valvular incompetence. The pressure and flow changes are basically different, but they take place simultaneously, which makes it very confusing. The physical environment in the veins determines the structure of the vein wall. A gradual increase in pressure produces hypertrophy, while a turbulent downward flow produces an asymmetrical, atrophic, bulging dilation that we recognise as a varicose vein. Valvular incompetence can be due either to dilation - it which case it is reversible - or to thrombosis and recanalisation - in which case it is irreversible. Advantage can be taken of reversible dilation in planning the treatment of varicose veins.

If we locate the incompetent lower perforators and close them with fibrosis, we then restore the pump efficiency and reduce the pressure in the superficial veins. This reduction in pressure allows the diameter of the superficial veins to reduce and the valves to recover their function. The restoration of normal pressure can cause even a saphena varix to return to normal. The location and induced fibrosis of perforating veins should be carried out as soon as possible to take advantage of the ability of veins to return to normal.

Superficial veins are quite different from deep veins in structure and function. The superficial veins are the auricles of the deep veins; they collect blood and store it until the deep vein pressure is low enough to receive it.

Flow and Pressure

There are four different pressures in the veins: the systolic pressure in the deep veins, the diastolic pressure in the deep veins, the hydrostatic pressure in the superficial veins, and the osmotic pressure of the plasma proteins.

The end result of the interplay of these pressures is to advantage the osmotic pressure in the plasma proteins and to allow absorption of tissue fluid. The site of this action is in the very small venules close to the capillaries that are devoid of muscle and are semipermeable. The arterial input in the tissues can be improved by improving the venous clearance in the capillaries and small veins. By cutting off the high pressure transmitted by the incompetent perforator, one can effect an improvement in venous clearance and arterial input. Arterial and venous ulcers are the result of inadequate perfusion. An ulcer is not the result of varicose veins and should not be called a varicose ulcer, any more than an arterial ulcer should be called a varicose ulcer. It is purely coincidental and not a sequester. Both arterial and venous ulcers are a failure of adequate perfusion, and the inadequate arterial input can be improved by improving the venous clearance. The abnormal flow in veins in the form of turbulent retrograde flow can be associated with good pumps, which have the ability to effect adequate venous clearance. Good pumps are associated with varicose veins but not with an ulcer. Varicosity in superficial veins is due to an abnormality of flow, while the venous ulcer is the result of the inability of the pumps to produce sustained low pressure after the commencement of walking. It is necessary to reduce the hydrostatic pressure below the osmotic pressure in order to advantage tissue fluid absorption. A favourable gradient between osmotic and hydrostatic pressure has to be maintained for the dialysis of the tissues and the prevention of ulcers.

The function of superficial veins is to collect, store and transmit blood from the skin to the deep veins. Superficial veins are, in effect, the auricles of the deep vein pumps. The effect of turbulence on the vein wall should be investigated more widely. There are many examples of its damaging effect, and it is easy to record this effect by the disappearance of muscle in the vein wall. It is quite common to see masses of varicose veins in legs with good pumps, and it would almost appear that we have to have good pumps in order to lift and leak enough blood after the commencement of walking. Increased velocity, reverse flow and turbulence in the medium-sized vein that is poorly supported by Sherman's fascia will produce varicosity, which will disappear when the abnormal flow is corrected.

The turbulent downward flow that takes place as a result of walking is thrashing against the wall of the semi-collapsed vein and can be compared to the turbulent flow from a high mountain stream. It is very different from the sluggish movement of blood in the standing patient, which is exemplified by the streams in the Everglades. The fact that veins are collapsible conduits suggests that it is possible to use the mountain stream and the Everglade swamps as analogous. Grass grows on the banks of the Everglades, but it does not grow alongside the fast-flowing mountain stream.

Location of Incompetent Perforating Veins

The success of the technique of compression sclerotherapy is dependent largely on the practitioner's ability to find and destroy incompetent valves in perforating veins.

The technique that I used depends on the outlining of the superficial veins in the standing patient by inspection, palpation and percussion. After outlining the superficial veins in the standing patient, the patient is then asked to lie down and the leg is elevated to empty all the blood out of the superficial veins; this takes a few minutes. When the leg is emptied, palpation of the leg reveals a very different limb from the standing limb. It is easy to palpate the bones, the fascia, the muscles, and any unsuspected thrombosed veins. This palpation reveals either holes or soft spots in the deep fascia surrounding the muscles; these points are marked with different coloured skin pencils. The tips of the fingers are pressed into these points, and the patient is asked to stand up; the fingers are then released one by one, moving from below upwards, and filling of the superficial complex reveals the presence of an incompetent perforator. The superficial veins related to these sites are the veins of choice for injection. One's knowledge of the anatomy of a patient's superficial and deep veins is, of course, basic. By this method, we will locate 50% of incompetent perforators. By the third visit, this will be a 90% success rate and better than can be achieved with the operated technique where we are limited to one attempt to locate and deal with the incompetent perforators.

Compression Bandaging

Bandaging is assumed to be within the competence of any doctor or nurse, but superb bandaging is an art. The compression applied by the superb bandaging is uniform but changes hourly with the change in the volume of the leg and is frequently inadequate compression to obliterate the vein. It is absolutely necessary to have localised specific compression by the bevelled rubber pads over the injected segments of the veins. One should observe the mark of the pad on the leg after the bandaging is removed as proof of the efficiency of the specific compression of the vein by the pad and bandage. Success of the technique depends on adequate, specific, uninterrupted and prolonged compression bandaging.

The technique depends on the fibroblasts (which normally does not enter the vein) to produce the necessary fibrosis after the intima is stripped. Fibroblasts do not appear in histological examination until the seventh day. It is followed by a blood supply from the outer periphery of the vein wall. This invasion of fibroblasts and their blood supply are the essential healing process of fibrosis. This produces the permanent fibrotic segment of vein that restores the leaking pumps and takes approximately six weeks. The end point of localised specific compression is indicated by the production of a hard, painless, cord-like vein. Areas of thrombosis indicate poor technique and poor bandaging.

Proprioceptive tactile palpation of the limb while bandaging is of great importance to the production of superb bandaging.

Walking

The time schedule of maturation of fibroblasts and osteoblasts is similar. Both mature rapidly as a result of walking, but walking also improves the peripheral pumps. The difference between the peripheral pumps and the central pump (the heart, which is working every minute of every hour of every day) is that the peripheral pumps work only while we walk. When we stand, we damage the peripheral pumps. Walking is an important adjunct to compression sclerotherapy. The help that the peripheral pumps give to the central pump is now beginning to be appreciated. An additional heart in the circulation, which is what we have if we walk regularly, is of great benefit to the dialysis of many other organs of the human body.

George Fegan

A Short History of the Treatment of Venous Disease

S. Sarin

The changes occurring in the lower limb due to disturbance of the normal blood flow in the veins have been the subject of many medical manuscripts. This chapter is a synopsis of the history of some of the methods of treatment of this condition, and it indicates how little some of the basic principles have changed.

The Hellenistic golden age gave rise to more scientifically oriented medical practice, with rejection of the notion that disease was the work of demons. In the works attributed to Hippocrates (460–377 BC), there are numerous references to varicose veins. Hippocrates believed that "when a varix is on the fore part of the leg and is very superficial or below the flesh, and the leg is black and seems to stand in need of having blood evacuated from it, such swellings are not by any means to be cut open, for generally large ulcers are the consequence of such incisions, owing to the influx from the varix. But the varix itself is to be punctured in many places as circumstances may indicate". Thus Hippocrates may have been the first person to note an association between ulcers and varicose veins and to recommend incision of the varices and compression to squeeze out the "humours".

The rise of the Roman Empire saw Aulus Cornelius Celsus in AD 30 deal with the treatment of ulcers by bandaging with linen. In the last two books of his *Eight Books on Medicine*, he also described the avulsion of varicose veins, although Galen (AD 130–200) is said to have expanded on these techniques. Galen's erroneous views of anatomy and physiology were based on comparative anatomical dissections (he had little access to human post-mortem specimens), and the dogmatic views of the Church marked an enduring stagnation in the development of surgery in Europe through the Middle Ages.

The advent of the Arab Empire ensured continued interest in the Greek school of medicine. Paul of Aegina (AD 607–690), a Byzantine surgeon, described mid-thigh ligation of the long saphenous vein (LSV) and postoperative bandaging long before Trendelenburg. He wrote:

> Varices of the leg may be operated upon in a manner similar to that for varicocele, making the attempt upon those in the inner part of the thigh where they generally arise, for below this they are divided into many ramifications. A tourniquet is placed upon the thigh and the patient walks. When the vein becomes distended a mark is made with writing ink or collyrium. Having placed the man in a reclining position with his leg extended we apply another tourniquet above the knee, and where the vein is distended we make an incision through the skin. The vein is freed and the tourniquets removed. A double thread is introduced under the vein and cut so as to make two ligatures, and the vein is opened in the

middle, and as much blood as is required is evacuated. The wound is dressed with a pledget in it and with an oblong compress soaked in wine and oil. It is then bandaged.

Two physicians, Ali bin Sina (later known as Avicenna; AD 981–1038) and Abul Qasim (also known as Albucassis; AD 936–1013), revived the old humoral ideas. Albucassis performed a type of internal stripping in the eleventh century using a needle and thread with a probe attached; after introduction of the needle, the probe was used to strip a section of vein. Ali bin Sina is said to have held the view that ulcers should not be allowed to heal, in order to allow the humours to escape. Both Ali bin Sina and Albucassis encouraged the use of bandaging with wine-moistened compresses. In the section on dermatology in the 20-volume *Al Malaki*, Ali bin al-Abbas (also known as Haly Abbas) in AD 994 stated: "Varicose veins are filling of the veins and their thickening, and they arise from a black bile mixture, which is poured into these veins and fills them, and they arise mostly in those who overwork their feet, and stand long on them, and through prolonged work of the body." It could be said, therefore, that by the eleventh century the major surgical principles of treatment of varicose veins were well outlined.

Henri de Mondeville (?–1320) described compression of the whole limb to "drive back the evil humours infiltrated in the leg and ulcer". This was the first challenge to the writings of Galen and marked the resurgence of European medicine and a return to the humoral school. In 1555 Marianus Sanctus of Barletta associated varicosities with childbearing, and Ambroise Paré (1510–1590) advocated mid-thigh ligation of varices and theorised that "heaping up" of suppressed menstruation during pregnancy was the cause of varicosities in women. The relaxation of the Church's ban on human dissection paved the way for the anatomists, with Leonardo da Vinci (1452–1519) producing over 779 anatomical drawings, many of which illustrated the venous system. The anatomist Vesalius (1514–1564) described the venous system in great detail but could not find the valves alluded to by Canano in 1546. However, both Fabricius (1537–1619) and Alberti publicly demonstrated venous valves, and the first illustration of a valve in a vein appeared in Alberti's book in 1585.

The concept of blood circulation is attributed to William Harvey (1578–1657), a student of Fabricius. Interestingly, a Spanish priest and doctor, Miguel Serveto (1511–1553), exiled in Vienna, considered blood to be the soul of the flesh. In one section of his book *Christianismi Restitutio*, he wonders whether blood is transferred from the pulmonary artery to the pulmonary vein during a passage through the lungs "while it is worked upon and keeps a light red colour". The religious text proved interesting reading to the indignant priests, and Serveto was burned at the stake for his heretical theology. William Harvey's *Exercitatio Anatomica de Motu Cordis et Sanguinis in Animalibus* (*An Anatomical Treatise on Heart and Blood Movement in Animals*) was published in 1628; using simple, fundamental observations, he concluded that blood circulated around the body.

These new concepts gave stimulus to the mechanical theories. Wiseman in 1676 re-described the association of varicose veins and ulceration, coined the term "varicose ulcer", and developed a laced compression stocking. Jean Louis Petit (1674–1750) stated that anything that caused an obstruction to the rising of blood in the veins was the principle cause of varicosities, while Dionis in 1708 attributed varicose veins in pregnant women to the pressure of the uterus on the iliac veins. Home (1756–1832) noted the importance of collateral vessels as a cause of recurrence after ligation. In 1824, Briquet suggested in his thesis that the calf muscle acted as a pump but understood that it caused blood to flow from the deep to the superficial systems via the communicating veins. Brodie in 1846 described his test of preventing reflux down the LSV by the application of digital pressure and felt that surgical treatment was inappropriate for varicosities because they were almost always followed by recurrence of the varicosities. Hodgson in 1851 thought of ulcers near the ankle as being intractable but easily cured when the varicose condition of the leg was relieved. He also believed that treatment of varicose veins made the surrounding veins varicose as they had to accommodate more blood flow. Verneuil in 1855 suggested that varicose veins were caused by incompetence of the deep veins, described valves in the communicating veins, and understood that they stopped blood flowing from deep to superficial veins. He also described varicosities in the deep venous system, but these were demonstrated to be normal soleal veins by le Dentu in 1867, who went on to describe the deep venous system in greater detail. In 1868, Gay and Spender, writing independently, suggested that ulceration was not a direct consequence of varicosities. They postulated that ulceration was caused by some other condition of the venous system, of which varicosities were also a complication. This "other" condition was thought to be obstruction of the deep veins, and they noted that ulceration could occur in the absence of varicose veins, providing there had been post-thrombotic damage to the deep veins. As regards the treatment of venous disease, Martin in 1878 described the use of India rubber bandages to produce sustained compression. Trendelenburg in 1890 re-described Brodie's test and also ligation of the LSV in the upper third of the thigh.

Christopher Ubren and his associates in 1656 are reputed to have been the first to introduce drugs intravenously. Using a metal tube, they injected opium into the veins of a dog. Similar injections were given to humans a few years later by J.D. Major and Casper Scott. However, it was not until the development of the hypodermic syringe by Francis Rynd in 1845 that treatment of varicose veins by injection sclerotherapy began to attract attention. Cassaignaic and also Debout in 1853 used injections of perchloride of iron and reported some success. Soule noted the development of inflammation and suppuration following perchloride of iron injections and recommended the use of compression to prevent dilation of the veins after injection. A solution of iodotannin was used by Panas, who reported suppuration in both his patients, and gangrene of the skin in one of them. In 1876, Weinlechner reported the healing of a varicose ulcer by the injection of iron perchloride into varicose veins in the region of the ulcer. As the popularity of injection sclerotherapy accelerated, a variety of solutions were used, including carbolic acid, 5% phenol, luargol solution, sodium salicylate, sodium carbonate, quinine, urethane and sodium morrhuate.

However, popularity was soon followed by discredit, when in 1933 Foxon published the results of a follow-up survey of injection treatment showing a recurrence rate of 63%. Other series, such as those of Howard, Jackson and Mahon in 1931 and of Oschner and Mahorner in 1939, reported equally alarming rates of recurrence. With advances in surgery and anaesthetics and the discreditation of injection sclerotherapy, treatment returned to surgical techniques.

The origin of LSV stripping probably dates from the works of Madelung in 1844, who used an incision along the entire length of the vein. Trendelenburg (1844–1924) popularised high ligation of the LSV, although his published results after this form of treatment admit a recurrence rate of 22%. With the wider application of anaesthesia, a variety of surgical techniques for treating varicose veins were introduced. Intraluminal stripping was described by Keller in 1905, and Mayo described extraluminal stripping of the LSV in the following year.

At the beginning of the twentieth century, surgery for venous disease was aimed at the superficial veins. The major conceptual advance was made by Homans in 1917, who classified venous pathology into primary (normal deep veins) and secondary (deep veins showing evidence of post-thrombotic damage). He attributed large, dilated veins to the effects of strain or dilation of the vein wall. He attributed small, thickened veins to phlebitis, and he described "crippling" of the venous valves. He noted patients with the latter to be much more resistant to treatment. He also described incompetence of perforating veins in a proportion of cases but stated that the deep veins never became varicose.

For surgical treatment, Homans advised complete excision of all varicose veins. He considered the Trendelenburg procedure alone, i.e. ligation of the saphenofemoral junction, to be inadequate because of the high recurrence rate of varicosities (60–70% after five years). In view of this, he advocated either division of the main saphenous trunk in several places (described by Schwartz) or full excision either through a long incision or by stripping. Where there was ulceration, Homans also emphasised the importance of removing all scar tissue down to and including the deep fascia. By this manoeuvre, all underlying incompetent perforating veins would also be ligated. The defect was then covered by a skin graft. For "post-phlebitic" varicose veins, he recommended in addition ligation of all perforating veins in the lower leg. To accomplish this, depending on the condition of the skin, Homans used the longitudinal incision described by Madelung, the "spiral cut" described by Rindfleisch, or multiple incisions based on the "garter" operation of Schede. Nevertheless, recurrence of ulceration was common.

The presence of incompetent perforating veins in close proximity to venous ulcers had been noted by Homans. In 1938, Linton described incompetence of "communicating" veins between the saphenous and deep venous systems found at operation in a series of 50 patients. He recommended the ligation of these incompetent veins at their origin beneath the deep fascia, and described three long incisions down the leg – medial, anterolateral and posterolateral – for adequate exposure. This was combined with ligation of the saphenous veins if they were incompetent, and, in a proportion of patients with deep vein reflux, he performed ligation of the superficial femoral vein. In 1953, after a two- to-five-year follow-up, Linton reported a 55% ulcer recurrence rate following ligation of the communicating veins and a 60% recurrence rate after concomitant ligation of the superficial femoral vein.

Also in 1953, Cockett and Elgan-Jones hypothesised that ulceration was purely a local problem. They described poor arterial supply to the gaiter region of the leg and proposed that this factor, combined with incompetent perforating veins in this area, led to regional hypoxia. They noted that the saphenous system had little to do with the venous drainage of the gaiter region and blamed this on the frequent recurrence of ulceration seen following ligation of the LSV. They also proposed that the deep fascia of the lower leg was an essential part of the calf muscle pump. Cockett described a long incision down the medial aspect of the lower leg with ligation of perforating veins as they emerged from the deep fascia.

By the 1960s, varicose veins per se were no longer blamed for the skin changes associated with chronic venous insufficiency. Incompetence of perforating veins as a consequence of deep vein thrombosis (DVT) was believed to be the central problem. This opinion is still held widely today. Cockett's (or Linton's) operation was performed enthusiastically over the next decade. Various different incisions have been described, but the principle remains the same. Good results continued to be reported, with ulcer recurrence rates of approximately 15%. Enthusiasm waned in the

1970s, however, due to reports of high recurrence rates of ulceration and poor wound healing. The latter proved to be a frequent complication necessitating lengthy periods of hospitalisation.

Many of the basic principles and techniques advocated in this book have been mentioned by other authors in the past – injection of sclerosant, compression bandaging, avulsion of varicose veins – and it is a sobering thought that recent advances in diagnosis and treatment are only fine-tuning the models developed over the centuries.

2 Applied Anatomy of the Veins of the Lower Limb

T.R. Cheatle

The reader approaching a text on the subject of sclerotherapy may be forgiven for wondering why it should be necessary to read through a revised account of human venous anatomy. Can the arrangement of the veins of the leg have changed much since the time of Gray, let alone since the last edition of this book? Does evolution happen that quickly?

No, but our ideas of which anatomical features are important in understanding the manifestations of venous disease do alter, and there has been some change of emphasis in our knowledge, or at least our beliefs, about the relationship between the two over the past 25 years. In part, this is driven by what is available to us as clinicians. Since the first edition of this book, the relative importance attached to perforating veins decreased initially as the importance of superficial venous system incompetence in ulceration became better appreciated and as disillusionment with the wound-related morbidity attached to the operations of Dodd and Cockett grew. The finding that in health blood can flow both ways in perforating veins also led to conceptual difficulties with the idea of incompetent perforators. Now, with the advent of subfascial endoscopic perforator surgery (SEPS), interest in the ablation, and consequently the anatomy, of perforating veins is re-emerging. It has been said, rightly, that the technical ability to perform an operation does not constitute an indication, but such technical advances do at least lead to a re-evaluation of an operation's worth.

Microcirculatory abnormalities in the skin of patients with venous disease are recognised increasingly as being of direct relevance to the clinical features of lipodermatosclerosis and ulceration. A short account of the microanatomy of the skin vasculature will therefore be given.

The deep and superficial fascia of the lower limb is concerned with the function of the veins and plays an important part in the action of the venous pumps. The relevant features will be described here.

General Features

Veins differ from arteries in a number of ways. Veins have thinner walls with very little muscle and are, as a result, both distensible and collapsible. Unlike arteries, veins can be divided into deep and superficial systems. Deep veins are very thin-walled and tend to be arranged in pairs accompanying the axial arteries (venae comitantes). Superficial veins have more muscle in their walls and tend to run singly, separated spatially from the arterial tree. The two systems are connected by perforating veins (so called because they perforate the fascia; some authors prefer the term "communicating veins" because their importance lies in the fact that they communicate between different compartments). Large veins are themselves drained by vasa venora, which can flow back into the parent vein, into other axial veins, or into the arterial system by small arteriovenous connections. The presence of the latter has long been a subject of debate in phlebology circles, but their existence is supported strongly by a recent micro-anatomical study by Crotty.

Arteriovenous Communications in Varicose Veins

Historically, the combination of increased pO_2 in the blood of varicose veins and a hyperdynamic circulation along with the supposed presence of venous stasis in the skin led to the concept that arteriovenous shunting was occurring in venous disease. There followed a prolonged search for abnormal arteriovenous communications.

Small arteriovenous connections (Sucquet–Hoyer canals) are almost certainly a normal feature in mammalian skin and form part of the thermoregulatory mechanism. These arteriovenous connections are microscopic; the vessels postulated as being responsible for the phenomena described above were of a different order of magnitude.

Gius claimed to identify abnormal arteriovenous communications entering the LSV in 13 patients undergoing varicose vein surgery. He traced these vessels to the tibial arteries in the subfascial compartment. Similar findings were reported by Piulachs and Vidal Barraquer and by Haeger and Schalin. These reports are hard to evaluate because the presence or absence of similar appearances in normal controls is difficult to ascertain in life.

Other evidence adduced to support the presence of such vessels included thermographic findings indicating that skin in legs with varicose veins was warmer than in normal legs. This was clearly very circumstantial evidence, as a number of alternative explanations are possible for this finding, including capillary proliferation, inflammatory hyperaemia, and autonomic dysfunction.

Rapid venous filling at arteriography has also been described in patients with varicose veins, but the arteriovenous fistulae supposedly responsible have not been seen radiologically.

The subject seems to have lapsed as a topic of active surgical research. Many surgeons accept the negative results of Partsch's group, who examined shunt volumes in normal controls and varicose vein patients using microspheres and found no demonstrable difference between them. They concluded that arteriovenous communications were not a haemodynamically significant factor in patients with varicose veins. The subject of arteriovenous shunts in venous disease has been reviewed by Scott (see *Further Reading*).

Flow through veins is directed by the presence of valves, which are of fundamental importance in the return of blood to the heart. Venous valves are bicuspid, consisting of two intimal folds on a thin collagenous supporting layer, lined on both sides by endothelium. The junction of cusp with vein wall is known as the agger. The agger is devoid of muscle in the jugular veins, but it has a well-developed muscle content in the saphenous veins. It has been suggested that this may reflect a degree of contractility at the valve level, possibly responding to changes in blood flow (the valves are not innervated). The lumen of the vein widens above the agger to form a sinus, an area of vortical flow and stagnation where most thrombi probably originate.

When venous pressure distal to a valve is greater than the pressure on the proximal side, the cusps are pushed open and blood flows towards the heart. When the pressure gradient is reversed, the cusps are held closed, preventing retrograde flow. Incompetence of the venous valves, due either to a congenital defect or to post-thrombotic destruction, allows retrograde flow, or reflux, to occur, with a variety of well-known pathological consequences.

Blood Supply to the Skin

Different descriptions of the circulatory arrangements within the skin abound. Much of the basic work in elucidating the anatomy of the skin circulation was done in the 1920s by Spalteholz in Germany. Generally, it is agreed that a number of different plexuses exist, but with a great degree of overlap and interconnection. These plexuses are arranged in strata throughout the dermis and are linked by vertical vascular channels.

The deepest of these is the "internal vascular belt" described by Moretti in 1968, which lies at the junction of the subcutaneous tissues and dermis. Vessels run vertically from this plexus through the reticular dermis before spreading out horizontally to form the subpapillary plexus. From here, capillary loops project into the papillae themselves and follow the course of the dermo-epidermal junction. In addition, there are individual plexuses around hair follicles and eccrine sweat glands. However, as Montagna and Ellis pointed out: "It will be noted that current studies place too much emphasis on the apparently predictable geometric distribution of cutaneous vessels. Although plexuses of sorts do exist, they are all interconnected by vessels which completely riddle the dermis."

Microscopic Structure of Skin Vasculature

At the microscopic level, a knowledge of some of the ultrastructural features of the skin capillaries is necessary for an understanding of many of the abnormalities seen in venous disease. Microcirculatory units in the skin, as elsewhere, comprise the precapillary arteriole, the capillary, and the post-capillary venule. Each capillary loop is approximately 0.2–0.4 mm in height. Capillary loops are found principally in the papillary portion of the dermis and project up the papillae towards the epidermis. The electron-microscopy studies of Yen and Braverman have yielded precise detail concerning the structure of these vessels.

Tracing the course of arterioles through the dermis, Yen and Braverman demonstrated that as the vessel diameter falls from approximately 30 μm to 15 μm, so it loses its muscular coat – the precapillary sphincter. The elastin layer, which normally lies between the muscular layer and the endothelium, thus becomes more peripheral, until it too is lost when the vessel tapers to less than 12–15 μm in diameter. Below this level, one is left with true capillaries composed of only an endothelial tube, a basement membrane, and occasional individual pericytes. Pericytes resemble poorly developed smooth-muscle cells, having less well-developed dense bodies, scattered cytoplasmic mitochondria, and fewer microfilaments. They form tight junctions with the endothelium through breaks in the basal membrane. The internal diameter of the capillary is 4–6 μm. Pinocytotic vesicles in both the endothelium and the pericytes are common. Weibal–Palade bodies, which contain von Willebrand factor, are scanty.

At the apex of the papilla, the endothelial cells become attenuated and the diameter of the capillary is at its narrowest. The gaps between individual endothelial cells are approximately 20 nm, but less on the luminal side, where the cells are apparently contiguous. Pericytes are scarce.

In the descending limb, the principal structural change involves the basement membrane. It becomes laminated; Yen and Braverman suggest that this structural appearance should be taken as representing the transition from capillary to post-capillary venule. Pericytes reappear, especially as the vessel leaves the papilla, and veil cells (fibroblasts) are also seen. Gradually, a thin, muscular coat develops (the ratio of luminal diameter to muscle coat thickness in these vessels is about 100 to one). Functionally, these vessels are of fundamental importance in the control of total resistance, capillary pressure and, hence, capillary filtration. They comprise the main part of the subpapillary plexus, where they are responsible for normal skin colour. From this plexus, larger venules run down through the reticular dermis into the internal vascular belt and on into the large collecting veins in the subcutaneous tissues.

The skin has been elucidated further by three-dimensional computer reconstruction from serial electron micrographs. These have shown more clearly than before the way in which the smooth-muscle cells of the terminal arteriole act as sphincters. They tend to have cytoplasmic "wings" that encircle the endothelial tube and often overlap one another. In the post-capillary venule, pericytes are shown to form large numbers of contact points with the endothelium, holding the venule in a vice-like grip. It is suggested that they may have a true contractile role to play in the determination of systemic resistance at this site, unlike in the larger venules, where they have fewer contact points and probably act as an architectural support.

It can be seen that the blood supply to the skin is greatly in excess of its nutritive requirement, especially when one considers that skin has one of the lowest metabolic rates of any organ. Temperature control is the generally accepted reason for the skin having this excessive blood supply, based on the presence of numerous arteriovenous shunts at the interface of the dermis and subcutaneous tissues. These communications, known as Sucquet–Hoyer canals, are muscular and under sympathetic innervation. They are particularly common in the feet, hands, lips, nose and ears; elsewhere, less specialised arteriovenous communications are found in lower numbers.

Under normal conditions, with only moderate sympathetic tone present, the shunts are at least partially open and there is free flow to the dermis, allowing heat radiation through the skin. In cold conditions, the shunts close under intense sympathetic stimulation; blood thus bypasses the dermis and heat is conserved. As the nutritive requirements of the skin are low, skin damage is unusual unless cold is prolonged and severe. Normal skin blood flow is approximately 250 ml/m^2/min; only when flow falls to below about 30 ml/m^2/min does skin damage follow. Conversely, in hot conditions the shunts are fully relaxed and flow to the skin is greatly increased, reaching values as high as 2 l/m^2/min. Thus, heart failure is commonly precipitated by hot weather as cardiac output increases.

The mechanism described above also indicates another benefit consequent upon the excessive vascularity of the skin. Sympathetic tone is increased in conditions of shock, e.g. hypovolaemic shock. By closing the shunts and by vasoconstricting the periphery, a considerable volume of blood is diverted to vital organs. Thus, the skin acts as a blood reservoir in a way that is analogous to the role of the spleen in dogs.

Special considerations apply to the situation in the leg. At birth, the lower-limb capillary pattern is the same in the leg as elsewhere. Ryan in 1970 pointed out that the disproportionate increase in limb growth compared with that in the face or trunk leads to an increase in skin surface area with which the dermal capillaries fail to keep pace, so the number of capillary loops in the skin of the leg is less than that in other sites. The capillaries themselves tend to be elongated and more convoluted than elsewhere, a change that is exacerbated in the presence of venous hypertension. Thus, even in health, there is a tendency towards uneven perfusion of the skin of the leg.

Veins of the Lower Limb

Figure 2.1 shows the main superficial and deep veins of the lower limb.

Veins of the Foot

The important veins of the foot are the deep veins of the sole, the superficial veins of the dorsum, and the perforating veins connecting them. The veins of the toes and the veins draining the superficial tissues of the sole are of no clinical significance.

The deep veins of the foot are the deep plantar venous arch and the medial and lateral plantar veins. The deep plantar venous arch runs from the proximal end of the first interosseous space, where it is continuous with the venae comitantes of the dorsalis pedis artery, across the foot to the base of the fifth metatarsal, accompanying the deep plantar arterial arch. It is a large vessel (up to 1 cm in circumference), and it receives the deep metatarsal veins and tributaries from the surrounding muscles. It is continuous at its lateral end with the lateral plantar veins, which run back across the sole accompanying the artery of the same name.

The medial plantar veins run from the medial end of the deep plantar venous arch along the medial edge of the sole to join the lateral plantar veins below the medial malleolus and form the posterior tibial veins. The plantar veins receive numerous tributaries from the surrounding muscles and from the superficial tissues of the sole. They have frequent valves, which allow only proximal flow of blood.

Emphasis has been placed recently on how the capacity of the deep veins of the foot is far in excess of that necessary to allow simple venous drainage of that appendage. Although not a new concept – Le Dentu first proposed it in 1867 – the idea that these veins act as a peripheral pump like a smaller version of the calf muscle pump has become established. Gardner and Fox covered the subject in detail (see *Further Reading*).

The superficial veins of the dorsum of the foot are the dorsal venous arch, the marginal veins, and the anterior vein of the leg. The dorsal venous arch lies over the proximal ends of the metatarsal bones and is usually visible. Its medial limb runs back along the medial side of the dorsum to become continuous with the LSV in front of the medial malleolus. The lateral limb lies along the lateral side of the dorsum, runs below the lateral malleolus, and becomes continuous with the short saphenous vein (SSV). The arch receives the dorsal metatarsal veins, the marginal veins, and tributaries from the superficial tissues of the sole. It is connected with the deep vessels by perforating veins, which are described below.

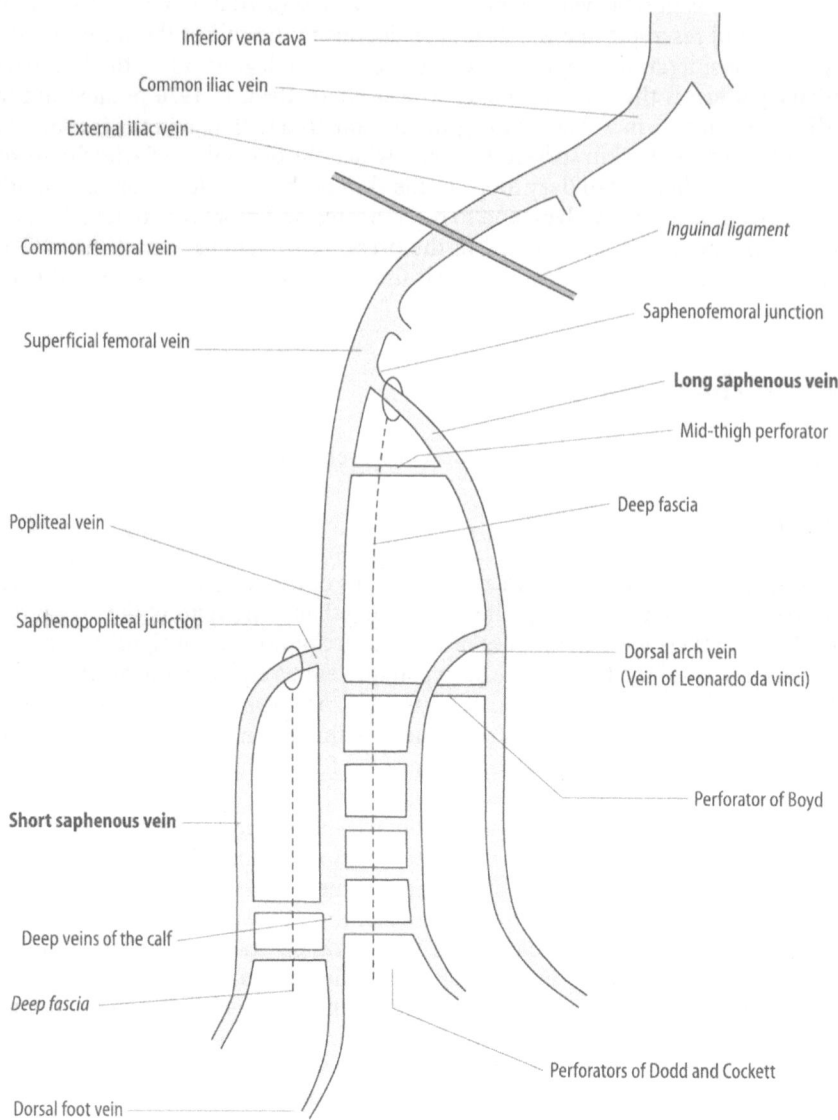

Figure 2.1 Anatomy of the venous system of the leg

The anterior vein of the leg arises from the distal part of the dorsal venous arch, runs back across the dorsum of the foot, and runs up the anterior aspect of the leg. Irregular vessels connect these superficial veins to form a network on the dorsum of the foot.

The perforating veins of the foot can be divided into two groups. The first group comprises those that connect the superficial veins with deep veins on the dorsum of the foot (the venae comitantes of the dorsalis pedis artery). Two of these are constant and connect the ends of the dorsal venous arch with the point at which the venae comitantes of the dorsalis pedis artery become continuous with the anterior tibial veins.

The second group comprises the perforating veins that connect the superficial veins with the deep veins of the sole. These are found at both margins of the foot and in the first interosseous space. There are usually five on the medial border of the foot, of which the most posterior is large and constant in site. This connects the junction of the medial and lateral plantar veins with the medial end of the dorsal venous arch, just in front of the medial malleolus.

A wide, constant, perforating vein at the proximal end of the first interosseous space connects the dorsal venous arch with the deep plantar venous arch. It accompanies the dorsalis pedis artery and veins into the sole. This vessel does not have a valve. On the lateral border of the foot, there are usually three perforating veins, of which one is constant. It is unvalved and runs from the lateral plantar veins alongside the tendon of peroneus longus to join the lateral marginal vein.

Deep Veins of the Lower Limb

The deep veins of the leg are the venae comitantes of the arteries (anterior and posterior tibial veins and the peroneal veins), the popliteal vein, and the intramuscular veins. The main deep veins of the thigh are part of the popliteal vein, the superficial and common femoral veins, and the profunda femoris vein. The venae comitantes are applied closely to their respective arteries, with frequent vessels joining the two veins and many valves allowing only proximal flow of blood.

The anterior tibial veins are the upward continuation of the venae comitantes of the dorsalis pedis artery. They accompany the anterior tibial artery to the upper border of the interosseous membrane, receiving tributaries from the muscles of the anterior compartment of the leg and several perforating vessels.

The posterior tibial veins are formed by the junction of the medial and lateral plantar veins below the medial malleolus. They run upwards beside the posterior tibial artery, between the superficial and deep groups of flexor muscles of the leg. They are joined by the peroneal veins, and then join with the anterior tibial veins at the lower border of popliteus to form the popliteal vein. They receive many tributaries from the surrounding muscles, especially the soleus, and the many perforating veins.

The peroneal veins arise from the posterolateral aspect of the calcaneum to run behind the inferior tibiofibular joint, and upwards along the course of the peroneal artery, between the flexor hallucis longus and the tibialis posterior. They receive tributaries from the surrounding muscles and perforating veins, and then join the posterior tibial veins 20–25 cm below the commencement of the popliteal vein.

The popliteal vein, formed by the union of the anterior and posterior tibial veins at the lower border of the popliteus, runs upwards through the popliteal fossa, crossing superficially from the medial to the lateral side of the popliteal artery. It is often duplicated, especially below the knee-joint line. It receives tributaries from the genicular plexus and from the surrounding soft tissues, including both heads of gastrocnemius, and is usually joined by the SSV.

The intramuscular veins of the leg are important because it is these vessels that make up the calf pump. The gastrocnemius is drained by a pair of venae comitantes from each head, which join the popliteal vein. The soleus muscle contains a variable number of wide, thin-walled veins, generally called sinuses, which run the length of the muscle. In the lower half of the leg, these drain by short vessels into the posterior tibial veins. The upper half of the soleus drains into both posterior tibial and peroneal veins. The deep flexor muscles are drained by short vessels that join the posterior tibial and peroneal veins at intervals.

These intramuscular veins are compressed and emptied when the muscles contract, providing the pumping action so important in venous return from the active limb. The vessels through which they empty into the venae comitantes of the arteries of the leg have valves allowing flow only in this direction.

Anatomy of the Gastrocnemius Veins

Being situated beneath the deep fascia of the leg, the gastrocnemius veins are part of the deep venous system. Within the muscle, they tend to run as straight leashes of heavily valved veins, amalgamating to form two main veins, one from each muscle head. These two either join the popliteal vein separately below the level of insertion of the SSV or occasionally drain into the SSV directly. This then usually empties into the popliteal vein as a common trunk, although, as is well recognised, the SSV is variable in its termination in about a third of all cases. Distally, the gastrocnemius veins often communicate with the superficial venous system via a mid-calf perforating vein at the so-called "gastrocnemius point" described by May and Nissl.

Hobbs has described the typical clinical features of gastrocnemius vein insufficiency. Patients complain of aching inside the calf on standing, often with a feeling of restlessness in the leg. There will usually be superficial varicosities, but these will always be posteriorly below the gastrocnemius point, i.e. below mid-calf. A venous flare may mark this point, and there may be a unilateral increase in calf girth.

The popliteal and femoral veins are frequently duplicated, forming a main channel running through a plexus. The profunda vein communicates with the femoral both below, where it joins the plexus in the adductor canal, and above the vessels, usually joining about 5 cm below the inguinal ligament. These veins receive tributaries from the surrounding muscles and perforating veins, of which the termination of the LSV is the largest.

The upper part of the popliteal vein comes to lie on the lateral side of the popliteal artery at the hiatus in the adductor magnus, where it becomes the femoral vein. This vessel crosses behind the femoral artery from lateral to medial in its course through the adductor canal and femoral triangle. The femoral vein may have up to six valves, but there are usually three, the commonest site being just distal to the point of entry of the profunda vein, and the second commonest site being at or just distal to the inguinal ligament. The first of these is the valve favoured by most surgeons for repair in patients with primary valvular incompetence.

Superficial Veins of the Lower Limb

The superficial veins of the leg are the long (great) saphenous and the short (lesser) saphenous veins, their tributaries, and the communicating veins connecting them. The LSV is the longest vein in the body. It commences in front of the tip of the medial malleolus, as the continuation of the medial limb of the dorsal venous arch of the foot. It runs upwards 2–3 cm in front of the tip of the medial malleolus, and then inclines posteriorly, crossing the medial surface of the tibia. It runs along the medial aspect of the leg to pass behind the medial condyle of the tibia into the thigh. It is applied closely to the saphenous nerve (L3 and L4), the largest cutaneous branch of the femoral nerve, which is sensory to the skin of the medial side of the leg down to and including the ankle. This nerve becomes subcutaneous by piercing the fascia lata between the heads of sartorius and gracilis, below which level it is particularly vulnerable to damage when the LSV is stripped below the knee.

The LSV has two main tributaries in the leg. The anterior vein of the leg, which has been described arising from the distal part of the dorsal venous arch of the foot, runs up the anterior aspect of the leg, 2–3 cm lateral to the anterior border of the tibia. At a variable level in the upper half of the leg, but usually just below the tibial tuberosity, it crosses the medial surface of the tibia and joins the LSV.

The posterior arch vein begins behind the medial malleolus, occasionally communicating with the constant most posterior perforating vein on the medial border of the foot. It runs upwards to join the LSV just below the knee.

The LSV enters the thigh behind the medial femoral condyle and then runs up the medial aspect of the thigh. It arches slightly forward to join the femoral vein at the saphenous opening, about 4 cm below and slightly lateral to the pubic tubercle. Its posteromedial tributary runs from the posterior aspect of the thigh, where it frequently communicates with the SSV, to join the LSV, usually at the level of the junction of the middle and upper thirds of the thigh, but sometimes as high as the saphenofemoral junction. The anterolateral tributary of the LSV begins at the lateral side of the upper leg, where it sometimes communicates with the lateral tributary of the SSV or the upper peroneal perforating vein. It runs upwards on the anterolateral aspect of the knee, and then runs obliquely across the anterior aspect of the thigh to join the LSV at any point between the midpoint of the thigh and the saphenous opening. In addition to the posteromedial and anterolateral tributaries, which may join the saphenous vein at the saphenofemoral junction, there are four smaller but more constant tributaries at this level that must be sought and divided during saphenofemoral disconnection for varicose veins. These are the superficial circumflex iliac vein, the superficial epigastric vein, and the superficial and deep external pudendal veins. The precise configuration of how these tributaries are related to the LSV is variable; it is not uncommon for the anterolateral or posteromedial tributaries to be as large as the LSV itself, or they may enter the femoral vein independently. Recognition of such anomalies is essential if varicose vein surgery is to be effective. The small external pudendal artery usually runs between the LSV and the superficial femoral vein about 1 cm below their junction, but occasionally it runs anterior to the LSV. It has no clinical significance and can be divided with impunity.

The average number of valves in the LSV is 8.7 (standard deviation [SD] 1–19). There are more valves in the thigh than in the leg. One valve, about 5 cm before the termination of the vein, is a constant feature and has been repaired by enthusiastic surgeons.

The SSV begins behind the lateral malleolus as the continuation of the lateral limb of the dorsal venous arch. It runs upwards along the lateral border of the Achilles tendon and, about halfway up the leg, pierces the deep fascia to run in the groove between the bellies of gastrocnemius. It is related closely to the sural nerve, which usually runs just lateral to the vein and is easily damaged if the SSV is stripped, although this risk has been reduced by the introduction of perforation/inversion (PIN) stripping.

In about three-quarters of cases, the SSV joins the popliteal vein in the popliteal fossa, diving between the bifurcation of the sciatic nerve to do so. It is much more variable in its termination than the LSV, a matter of importance surgically when one attempts saphenopopliteal disconnection. Pre- or peroperative imaging, by either duplex imaging or phlebography, is highly desirable in order to define the precise configuration.

In a phlebographic study, Lea Thomas and Chan found that only 61% of SSVs had a conventional termination with the popliteal vein in the popliteal fossa, and many of these lay up to 7.5 cm above the level of the joint line. In the remainder of cases, the SSV does not join the popliteal vein. In two-thirds of these, it joins deep or superficial vessels in the thigh – very occasionally in the buttock; in the remaining cases, it joins deep veins below the popliteal fossa.

Dodd described a "popliteal area" vein that drains the superficial tissues over the popliteal fossa and the adjoining parts of the back of the thigh and leg. It pierces the deep fascia in the centre of the fossa or at one of its corners (usually in the centre or at the lateral corner) to join the short saphenous, popliteal or gastrocnemial veins.

There are usually two or three communicating veins that run upwards and medially to join the posterior arch vein, with valves that allow blood to flow only in this direction. A tributary of the SSV runs up the posterolateral aspect of the leg, over the line of fusion of the posterior intermuscular septum with the deep fascia. It joins the SSV in the upper part of the leg and often communicates with the anterolateral tributary of the LSV, just below the neck of the fibula. A communicating vein joining the LSV and the SSV is often referred to as the "vein of Giacomini", but it is by no means a constant feature.

There are usually 7–11 valves in the SSV, allowing only proximal flow.

Perforating Veins of the Leg

The perforating veins of the leg all have valves that allow blood to flow only from the superficial to the deep veins. Typically, they are associated not with the saphenous veins but with their tributaries, and they may be divided conveniently into four groups according to the deep veins with which they are connected.

The anterior tibial group of perforating veins connects the anterior vein of the leg with the anterior tibial veins. There is a variable number, from three to ten. Some pierce the deep fascia at the anterior border of the tibia, some pass between the tibialis anterior and extensor digitorum longus, and others pass along the anterior intermuscular septum. Three are constant. The lowest is at the level of the ankle joint; the second is about halfway up the leg and has been called the "midcrural vein"; the third is at the point at which the anterior vein of the leg curves medially to cross the anterior border of the tibia. For the purposes of recording diagnosis, the inconstant perforating veins in this region can be divided into upper, middle and lower groups, in their respective thirds of the leg. The upper and lower perforators described here correspond to the veins of Cockett and Boyd, respectively.

The posterior tibial perforating veins connect the posterior arch vein with the posterior tibial veins, running in the transverse intermuscular septum. They can be divided into upper, middle and lower groups; there are usually five or six. In the upper group, there are one or two veins, piercing the deep fascia just behind the medial border of the tibia. The middle group is found in the middle third of the leg, the veins piercing the deep fascia 1–2 cm behind the medial border of the tibia; at least one of this group is always present. The lower group is found in the lower third of the leg; there are usually three or four, the lowest of which pierces the deep fascia 2–3 cm behind the lower border of the medial malleolus; another pierces the deep fascia 5–6 cm above this, and there are one or two more above this; the highest vein in this group lies at the junction of the middle and lower thirds of the leg.

On the posterior surface of the leg there is a group of soleal perforating veins, so called because they join the veins of the soleus and gastrocnemius muscles. There are usually three – upper, middle and lower – and these typically leave the communicating veins joining the SSV to the LSV, rather than the SSV itself. They may, however, arise somewhat lateral to the SSV, connecting either with it or with one of its small tributaries.

The peroneal group of perforating veins is found along the line of fusion of the deep fascia with the posterior intermuscular septum. There are usually three or four. Two are constant, one just below the neck of the fibula and the other at the junction of the middle and lower thirds of the leg, called the lateral ankle perforating vein. The others are very variable in position and may be divided into upper, middle and lower groups. These veins arise from the lateral tributary of the SSV, which ascends close to the line along which those veins pierce the deep fascia. They run to join the peroneal veins, along the posterior intermuscular septum.

Veins of the Thigh

The superficial veins of the thigh are the LSV and its tributaries. The most constant perforating veins in the thigh connect the LSV with the femoral vein in (Hunter's) adductor canal, and are therefore called the upper, middle and lower Hunterian perforating veins. The upper one pierces the roof of the adductor canal at its upper end. The middle one, which is constant, passes behind the sartorious to join the femoral vein. The lower Hunterian perforating vein pierces the deep fascia just above the medial femoral condyle to join the genicular venous plexus. This group of veins is sometimes also referred to as Dodd's veins.

There are three other perforating veins in the thigh, which appear sufficiently often to deserve mention. Two are connected with the anterolateral tributary of the LSV, at points where vertical lines drawn upwards from the margins of the patella cross it. These vessels join the tributaries of the lateral circumflex femoral vein. At the point at which the posteromedial tributary of the LSV crosses the tendons of semi-membranosus and semi-tendinosus, there is frequently a perforating vein that joins the profunda vein.

All of the perforating veins of the thigh have valves that allow blood to flow only from superficial to deep veins.

Fascia of the Lower Limb

Both the superficial and the deep fascia appear to be of importance in relation to venous return from the lower limb.

The superficial fascia shows two distinct layers. The superficial layer is of loculated fatty tissue, while the deep layer is a strong membrane of collagen, with some elastic tissue. The deep layer is defined particularly clearly in the foot, where it lies superficial to the dorsal venous arch and its tributaries but deep to the anterior vein of the leg. This deep layer of superficial fascia extends up the leg and thigh, covering the LSV and the SSV. The functional boundary between the superficial and deep veins is the deep fascia, and the membranous layer that lies over the main superficial veins should therefore be regarded as part of the superficial fascia.

The superficial fascia is homologous with Scarpa's fascia of the anterior abdominal wall, and these two fascial layers may be considered as a single continuous sheet, fused with the deep fascia of the thigh at the skin flexure crease of the hip joint, which is the lower limit of Scarpa's fascia. The structure of the two parts of this fascia is similar, containing a considerable quantity of elastic fibres.

The superficial veins can be divided into two groups, according to their relationship with the deep layer of superficial fascia. Deep to this layer lie the dorsal venous arch and both saphenous veins, and superficial to it lie the tributaries of the saphenous veins. It is of interest that throughout the limb, the veins that lie beneath the deep layer of superficial fascia show considerably less tendency to become varicose than those that lie superficial to it. The main trunk of the LSV is often dilated only moderately even when its tributaries are grossly varicose. In the foot, the anterior vein of the leg is commonly varicose when the dorsal venous arch remains normal.

These findings suggest that a function of the deep layer of superficial fascia is to give tangential support to the main veins of the lower limb. This would appear to be particularly important in the foot, where the dorsal venous arch is subjected to the pressures generated in the deep plantar veins.

The deep fascia of the lower limb is the functional boundary between deep and superficial veins. Askar and Abou-el-Ainen in 1963 described it as two layers, the superficial layer forming the crural fascia, which continues upwards to form the roof of the popliteal fossa, and the deep layer forming a layer over the muscles and continuing over the heads of gastrocnemius to join the femoral condyles. The deeper layer is really epimysium. Since the deep fascia surrounds the muscles of the limb and is relatively inextensible, contraction of the muscles causes a rise in pressure in the fascial compartments in which they lie. This pressure is exerted on the deep veins and provides the driving force in the calf muscle pump.

Another action by which the deep fascia may actively squeeze the leg rather than passively prevent it from expanding has been suggested by Askar. The fibres of the deep fascia on the posterior aspect of the leg form a diagonal lattice. Into the upper corners of this lattice are inserted extensions of the tendons of the hamstring muscles, which, when they contract, make the fascial tube longer and narrower. This reduction in diameter will compress the deep veins, aiding in the pumping action of the posterior compartment of the leg.

Conclusion

The descriptions of the deep and superficial veins of the lower limb given in this chapter are brief because variations in the anatomical arrangement are so common that constant features are few. Similarly, the number of perforating veins described is small. Those mentioned are vessels that occur sufficiently frequently and that are involved in varicose disease often enough for a knowledge of their usual sites and connections to be useful. As for the others, van Limborgh lists 214, which shows that perforating veins may be found almost anywhere in the limb. Knowledge of the anatomy is not a shortcut to diagnosis: it merely makes the diagnosis more meaningful. Careful examination of the whole limb is essential if all incompetent perforating veins are to be found.

3 Applied Physiology of the Veins of the Lower Limb

C. Rogers

The principle mechanisms that maintain venous return and the derangements that result in varicose veins are still understood incompletely. This is because veins, especially those of the dynamic lower limb, are extremely difficult to study. Their anatomy, pressure changes, and flow characteristics are highly variable and are susceptible to many local external influences. Since, pulmonary embolism apart, there are no obvious fatal venous diseases, research into venous pathophysiology has lacked the impetus behind that of arteries. In view of this relative neglect, the venous system has been called "the Cinderella of the circulation".

Although varicose veins occur rarely in quadrupeds, the adoption of the erect posture by *Homo sapiens* is undoubtedly the primary factor that predisposes to their development. Considerable effort has therefore been devoted to the study of venous pressure, especially in the upright posture. It should be remembered, however, that veins are not merely passive capacitance vessels. They are dynamic structures, and their primary function is to maintain venous flow. It is likely that increased understanding of the normal effects of blood flow and the perturbations that occur with altered anatomy will resolve the continuing debate about the aetiology of varicose veins.

Functional Anatomy

Venous structure is adapted especially to its function. Veins have the same basic three-layered structure as all blood vessels (with the exception of capillaries), consisting of an innermost tunica intima surrounded by a muscular tunica media and an outermost tunica adventitia. The tunica intima consists of flat endothelial cells resting on a thin connective tissue layer. The endothelial layer is mechanically weak and is destroyed easily by chemical and physical insults. Endothelial cells, however, demonstrate a marked capacity for regeneration and secrete many vasoactive products.

The tunica media consists of a spiral arrangement of spindle-shaped smooth-muscle cells within a matrix of elastin and collagen fibres. It supplies the mechanical strength and contraction power governing venous tone. The amount of smooth muscle in lower-limb veins increases from proximal to distal, with a thicker muscle coat in veins in the foot compared with those in the thigh. This enables distal veins to withstand greater hydrostatic pressures than proximal veins. The boundaries of the media are marked by internal and external elastic laminae.

The adventitia is a connective tissue sheath that merges with its surround. The elastin and collagen supply passive elasticity and resist distension.

Venous filling is dependent upon the distending pressure and the compliance of the vessel wall. The distending pressure is the transmural pressure (i.e. the intraluminal pressure minus the extraluminal pressure). The normal vein is elliptical in cross-section, with the short axis perpendicular to the skin.

When held above heart level, the transmural pressure decreases below zero and the vein collapses into a dumbbell shape with flow confined to the marginal channels. If the limb is lowered, the intraluminal pressure increases. As this pressure rises towards 10 cm H_2O, the elliptical profile becomes progressively more circular and the resistance to blood flow decreases.

Until the cross-section becomes circular, the vein can accommodate large volume changes without a significant increase in distending pressure. Further increases in volume are associated with a disproportionate increase in pressure, i.e. the pressure volume curve has reached its plateau. Maximum distensibility occurs at approximately 4 mm Hg and is estimated to be 100 ml/mm Hg for the human venous system. This is over 50 times greater than the compliance of the arterial system.

Above 10–15 cm H_2O, the profile is fully circular, and since the stretched collagen in the wall is relatively inextensible any further addition of even small volumes of blood (e.g. by calf muscle pump leakage through incompetent communicating veins) causes a significant increase in the superficial venous pressure. Normal veins are capable of withstanding pressures in excess of anything they may be called upon to endure.

The quantity of blood within the legs is therefore a function of body position. When erect, 300–800 ml of extracellular and vascular fluids (the quantities vary according to the experimental method and size of the subject measured) collects in the legs. This includes a 15% increase in blood volume. The venous system, especially in the legs, is therefore an important component of the cardiovascular system's circulatory reservoir. Much of this capacity is located in the numerous venules and small veins of diameter 20 μm–4 mm.

Valves

The direction of venous blood flow is controlled by the semilunar valves. Venous valves are bicuspid, with their free edges parallel to the skin's surface. Even though they consist of just a thin layer of collagen fibres covered with endothelium, the valves are extremely strong.

The distribution of the valves in the veins of the lower limb has been demonstrated by numerous cadaver dissection studies. The inferior vena cava, the common iliac vein, and 75% of external iliac veins have no valves. Below the inguinal ligament, the number of valves in each segment increases steadily so that the calf veins have valves that are 5 cm apart. Valves are present in veins of 1 mm diameter but not in smaller veins or venules. The valves in the communicating veins of the calf stop blood flowing from the deep to the superficial veins, but most of the valves in the communicating veins of the foot point in the opposite direction.

Valve function is not solely the result of cusp movement. It is a complex change involving valve sinus distension, which tightens the edges of the cusps by separating the commissures. Because of the spiral disposition of the elastic fibres and smooth muscle, circumferential strips of vein are slightly less elastic than longitudinal strips. By contrast, circumferential strips from the valve sinus are more elastic. This enables the sinus to balloon out more easily and turn the combined cavities of the two valve sinuses into a sphere.

If this does not happen, due to a lack of vein distensibility or elongation of the free edges of the cusps, the valve cusps may prolapse, leading to incompetence. Therefore, for valvular damage to occur, the vein diameter must first dilate to render the valves incompetent. When competent, venous valves can withstand pressures of up to 3 atm.

The complexity of the whole valve structure suggests that the valve may be able to open and close actively in response to circulatory demand. The peculiar construction of the cusp suggests that it possesses the ability to ruche up when the vein contracts. The electron microscope demonstrates that the endothelium is disposed longitudinally on the luminal aspect of the valve cusp in continuity with the endothelial lining of the vein while it runs transversely on the sinus aspect of the valve.

Venous Tone

In 1669, Richard Lower used the phrase "relaxato venarum tono" in his book *De Corde*. This was the first description of venous tone. Venous tone has an effect on the rate of blood flow, but it is involved more in the distribution of blood throughout the body. Active tone is provided by the smooth muscle in the tunica media. Passive tone is provided by the elastic properties of the vessel wall. At rest, most veins, especially the large collecting deep veins, have little active tone. Changes in tone are mediated through the sympathetic system controlled from the brainstem and spinal reflexes. In addition to the pressor and depressor areas, an important thermoregulatory area exists in the brainstem that controls the tone of the subcutaneous veins. Venous tone in the limb is determined further by locally released neurohumoral mediators and factors expressed within the vein wall (Table 3.1).

Table 3.1 Factors responsible for alterations in venous smooth-muscle tone

	Venoconstriction	Venodilation
Adrenergic	Emotion/pain	Sleep
	Deep breath	Local hyperthermia
	Exercise	Elevated core temperature
	Standing upright	
	Valsalva manoeuvre	
	Mental arithmetic	
Humoral	Noradrenaline	Phenoxybenzamine
	Adrenaline	Phentolamine
	Acetylcholine*	Reserpine
	Prostaglandins**	Barbiturates
	Histamine	Anaesthetics
	Serotonin	Alcohol
Vein wall	Endothelin	Nitric oxide
		Prostacyclin

*Acetylcholine can cause both constriction and relaxation. **Most prostaglandins dilate the valves but some cause constriction.

Veins have an adrenergic innervation through nerve endings that terminate in the tunica media. The density of nerve endings varies: the cutaneous veins have a rich innervation, whereas the veins in the skeletal muscles have few endings and so share a minimal response to sympathetic stimulation. Venodilation is normally achieved through a reduction in adrenergic tone, provided this is present. Overall, the most important reflex role of the subcutaneous veins is in thermoregulation. The veins also respond to local stimuli. A direct injury causes venospasm. Conversely, venospasm may be overcome by repeated, gentle, blunt trauma, e.g. tapping with the finger.

Myelinated nerve fibres exist in the vein wall; these fibres are involved in the perception of pain and detecting changes in temperature and pressure stretch reflexes. Since the outermost media and adventitia contain the nerve endings, myogenic conduction contributes to the neurogenic activation by coordinating venous contraction. Even in the outer layers of the media the separation of muscle cells from nerve endings is rarely less than 1000 Å. Therefore, an intact smooth-muscle layer is important in vein physiology.

By contrast with the subcutaneous veins, intramuscular veins are poorly innervated. Their volume is influenced chiefly by body posture (i.e. gravity) and the muscle pump. Although direct sympathetic control of these veins is almost non-existent, their volume is, nevertheless, affected indirectly by adrenergic activity because arteriolar constriction reduces the downstream pressure, allowing the venous system to recoil elastically.

Veins respond in the same way as arterioles to many stimuli, but there are some differences. Most veins have little basal tone in the absence of sympathetic activity and, except for the portal vein, they show little myogenic response to stretch. Angiotensin has little direct effect on veins, but it does act indirectly via the sympathetic nerves to potentiate the effect of adrenergic stimulation on human veins (neuromodulatory action). This contributes to the intense venoconstriction seen in patients with cardiac failure. Histamine causes veins to constrict but causes arterioles to dilate. The efficacy of glyceryl trinitrate in relieving angina is due partly to the reduction of cardiac preload due to the greater dilatory effect on veins than on arterioles.

Endothelium

Originally regarded as a selective but essentially passive permeability barrier between circulating blood and extravascular tissues, it is now recognised that endothelial cells possess a wide repertoire of active functions that are concerned with the regulation of vascular homeostasis. The endothelium therefore not only provides an anti-thrombotic lining but also produces a variety of substances, including nitric oxide, endothelin, prostacyclins, platelet-activating factor, von Willebrand factor, tissue plasminogen activator, and a number of cytokines, growth factors and leucocyte adhesion molecules. Endothelial cells can therefore regulate vascular tone, vessel-wall permeability, haemostasis, coagulation and fibrinolysis, and interactions with leucocytes.

In 1980, Furchgott and Zawadski discovered that whereas a normal artery ring relaxes in response to acetylcholine, when the endothelial lining is removed the response changes to constriction. The response to several potent in vivo vasodilators (adenosine triphosphate [ATP], bradykinin, acetylcholine) in human hand veins changes to constriction if the endothelial lining is destroyed by local perfusion with distilled water. Arterial and venous endothelium synthesises a vasodilator substance, initially called endothelium-derived relaxing factor (EDRF), in response to stimulation by acetylcholine. EDRF diffuses directly from the endothelial lining into the underlying vascular smooth muscle, activating the enzyme guanylyl cyclase and initiating a rise in cyclic guanosine monophosphate (cGMP), which induces venous smooth-muscle relaxation.

EDRF is now known to be nitric oxide, which is synthesised from L-arginine and has a half-life of approximately six seconds. Nitric oxide production is also stimulated by a number of other substances, such as thrombin, bradykinin, histamine, serotonin and ATP, and by altered shear.

Endothelial cells also produce vasoconstrictor substances. Recently discovered endothelin (ET-1) causes a strong vasoconstriction in arteries lasting several hours. Its physiological role in veins is still under investigation. In both arteries and veins it appears that nitric oxide can inhibit constriction to endothelin. Arteries release more nitric oxide than do veins, and the effects of nitric oxide are reduced by endothelium-derived elements originating from the cyclo-oxygenase pathway. However, venous smooth muscle is more sensitive than arterial smooth muscle to both nitric oxide and endothelin. Therefore, the lower basal release of nitric oxide is more effective in veins than in the corresponding arteries and contributes to the greater sensitivity of the venous circulation to nitrates.

Many of the agents that induce nitric oxide synthesis in endothelial cells also stimulate the release of prostacyclin. Endothelial cells are the most important source of prostacyclin, which, in addition to its powerful antiplatelet action, is a potent vasodilator.

The endothelial cells of the veins are a major source of fibrinolytic activator. The existence of a system opposed to coagulation has been known for many years. Todd established its site of production when he demonstrated that slices of veins incubated on fibrin plates caused areas of fibrinolysis. The presence of this fibrinolytic activity derived from the venous endothelium led Feamley to propose the concept of "natural fibrinolysis".

Normal lower-leg veins are unable to produce as much fibrinolytic activator as arm veins, and there is a relationship between venous pressure and activator release. Changes in vein-wall configuration, intraluminal pressure, shear stresses, and tension all affect the capacity of the endothelium to secrete its products. This adds a further dimension to the difficulties in understanding the effects of disordered circulation in varicose veins.

Gravity

In 1758, Sharp demonstrated in his book *A Treatise on the Operations of Surgery* an appreciation that gravity affects blood flow. Many textbooks on venous physiology often start with the principle that venous return from the lower limb in the erect posture must overcome gravity. This assumption is incorrect, since it ignores the fact that gravity has an equal effect on the arterial column. The pressure difference between arteries and veins at any vertical level, therefore, is not altered directly by orthostasis. Neither, therefore, is blood flow. The circulation through the limb resembles flow through a U-tube. Indeed, if blood vessels were completely rigid, then gravity would have no overall effect on the circulation. The adoption of a standing position increases the pressure in all blood vessels below heart level and reduces it in those above, because gravity acts on the column of blood between the heart and the vessel. Although this applies equally to arteries and veins, it is particularly noticeable in the latter since they have thinner, more compliant and, consequently, more distensible walls.

Tilting a human subject upright results in a transitory closure of the venous valves in the limbs. This prevents any significant retrograde flow of blood away from the heart. Pressure in the dependent veins then rises steadily over approximately 30-60 seconds because blood continues to flow into the veins from the arterial system. This increased volume is accommodated by the more compliant vein walls. As the intraluminal pressure rises, it will equal and then exceed that above the venous valves, which therefore open. This re-establishes an uninterrupted column of blood between the heart and the feet. The venous pressure in the feet increases tenfold, from approximately 10 mm Hg supine to nearly 100 mm Hg upright. With no counterbalancing rise in extramural pressure, the veins distend. This is plainly visible in one's own hand on lowering it below heart level.

In an adult human, about 500 ml of extra blood accumulates over 45 seconds in the distended veins of the lower limbs. This is usually called "venous pooling". Most of this blood comes ultimately from the intrathoracic compartment, causing the central venous pressure (CVP) to fall and, occasionally, dizziness or fainting to occur. This affect is pronounced if the subject is warm (venodilated) and standing motionless (e.g. standing to attention on military parade).

Limb blood flow does, in fact, decrease with dependency because of arteriolar constriction, which occurs as a reflex response to the orthostatically induced fall in cardiac output and to the rise in local transmural pressure. The latter response was first described by Sir Williams Bayliss, brother-in-law of Ernest Starling, in 1902. The myogenic response safeguards arterial blood flow and capillary filtration in the face of blood pressure alterations but, apart from the portal mesenteric vein, appears to be absent in veins.

Furthermore, gravity influences the formation and reabsorption of tissue fluids. Rising from supine to a passive standing position initially causes a dramatic increase in capillary pressure (Pc) in the feet. If vascular resistance remained unchanged, then capillary pressure would rise by 90–110 mm Hg, depending on the height of the individual. Fortunately, the rise in Pc is diminished greatly by local vasoconstriction, which may be partly myogenic and partly a local axon reflex involving sympathetic nerves. Even so, Pc reaches approximately 95 mm Hg in the motionless dependent foot and exceeds plasma colloid osmotic pressure (Pic) throughout most of the lower body in the upright position.

Prolonged standing in normal subjects results in swelling around the ankles, suggesting that there is a favourable gradient for the formation of interstitial fluid. Physiology textbooks traditionally depict fluid flux at the microcirculatory level according to the Landis–Starling model, which excludes the extravascular forces (interstitial pressure, Pii, and oncotic pressure, Pi) (Figures 3.1 and 3.2). The validity of the Starling principle of fluid exchange has been confirmed repeatedly, but the question of how transcapillary pressures and flows actually balance along a capillary in vivo has proved much more elusive. Landis's experiments were performed with tissues bathed in a protein-free saline bath, which causes Pii and Pi to be near zero. The extravascular Starling pressures (Pii and Pi) are therefore smaller than the

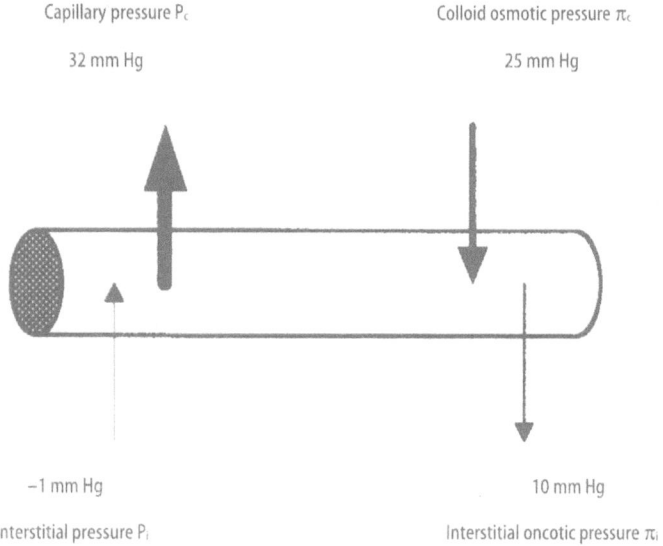

Capillary pressure P_c

32 mm Hg

Colloid osmotic pressure π_c

25 mm Hg

−1 mm Hg

Interstitial pressure P_i

10 mm Hg

Interstitial oncotic pressure π_i

Figure 3.1 Classical Starling's forces at the arterial end of the capillary.

intravascular pressures (Pc and Pic) and are often omitted from introductory text-books on the basis that they are negligible.

If these pressures are taken into account, then it can be shown that well-perfused systemic capillaries are commonly in a state of filtration over their entire length. Transient absorption may occur following vasoconstriction, but it cannot be maintained since Pii would increase and Pi would decrease. These changes would therefore abolish the net absorptive force and absorption would fade with time. Landis, in his classic experiment in 1927, presumably observed only the transient state of absorption at low capillary pressures rather than the steady state observed by Michel and Phillips in 1987.

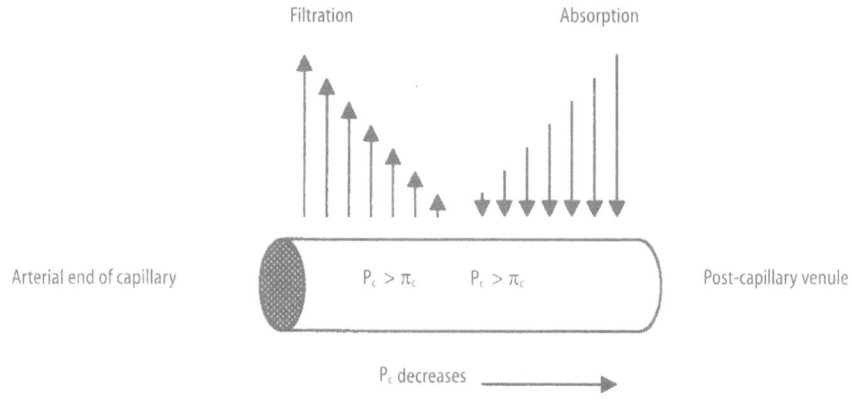

Filtration   Absorption

Arterial end of capillary $P_c > \pi_c$ $P_c > \pi_c$ Post-capillary venule

P_c decreases

Figure 3.2 Landis–Starling diagram. Net flux of fluid indicates filtration at the arterial end, equilibration at the midpoint, and reabsorption at the venous end (ignores **Pii** and pi).

If net fluid flux across the capillary is filtration without reabsorption, then the end result would be accumulation of fluid in the interstitium, i.e. oedema. In healthy individuals, this does not normally occur. There must, therefore, be a mechanism for interstitial fluid to be returned to the circulation. This is provided by the lymphatic system.

Lymphatic System

Virtually all tissues form lymph. This proves that there is a net filtration of fluid out of the microcirculation. There is increasing evidence that lymphatics function as a series of pumps that empty by active contraction of the lymphatic wall. Anchoring filaments assist in re-expansion of the terminal lymphatic, and intralymphatic pressure drops transiently below that of the interstitium, thus setting up a pressure gradient.

Once formed, lymph is propelled by intrinsic rhythmic contractions with a typical rate of 10–15 ml/min. Extrinsic propulsion by intermittent compression (during movement) increases lymph flow and is important for non-contractile vessels, such as those in the mesentery. The valves permit pressure to rise stepwise in successive segments, so that lymph finally drains into venous blood at several millimetres of mercury above atmospheric pressure.

The lymphatic circulation used to be estimated as 2–4 l/day in the adult. This estimate was based on the collection of lymph from accidental thoracic duct fistulae and has recently been revised because thoracic lymph is efferent lymph that has already passed through one or more groups of lymph nodes. Systemic nodes can alter the volume of lymph as it passes through them. Thus, given a postnodal flow of 4 l/day in humans, it is likely that the true extracapillary fluid circulation could be 8 l/day or more, of which 4 l is reabsorbed directly into the bloodstream by the lymph node microcirculation.

With advancing age, there is loss of elasticity of the tissues. The filaments anchoring terminal lymphatics are stretched, and the blind lymphatic requires a greater hydration in the interstitium to tighten these filaments. Interstitial fluid reabsorption is therefore disturbed at the very site of lymph formation. Any chronic oedema may stretch these anchoring filaments, and this may be one reason why chronic oedemas become refractory to treatment. Finally, this may be the cause of the well-known problem in clinical medicine of an inexplicable, more or less permanent swelling of the legs in otherwise healthy individuals.

Pumps

Heart

In a supine position, blood flows evenly along all superficial and deep vessels towards the heart. The heart acts on the venous return by two effects: vis a tergo is the positive pressure that is transmitted from the capillaries to the venous bed; vis a fronte represents the sucking action of the right atrium on the venous system. The pressure at the venous end of the capillary at heart level (12 mm Hg) increases by almost the full hydrostatic pressure effect below heart level. Thus, vis a tergo is responsible for the maintenance of the constant supply of blood to the venules in the lower limb. It has been suggested that minor variations in tone assist venous return by an effect on the vis a tergo when the other mechanisms of venous return are at a low ebb.

The presence of the vis a fronte factor has been demonstrated in open-chest animals. The end result of its action is a reduction in the pressure in the vena cavae. Since the establishment of a pressure gradient promotes flow to the area of the lower pressure, the vis a fronte contribution should theoretically assist central flow. In humans, this contribution is negligible. The atrial pressure pattern in the thoracic inferior vena cava disappears almost immediately below the diaphragm, and the vis a fronte effect is not detectable in any of the major intra-abdominal veins in erect and horizontal subjects.

Skeletal Muscle Pump

In his second book, *Tractatus de corde*, Lower clearly appreciates the effect of the limb muscles on blood flow, thus providing the first description of the peripheral venous muscle pump. In 1824, Briquet wrote a detailed thesis on venous disease. He understood that the calf muscles acted as a pump, but he thought that all blood flowed out of the lower limb through the superficial veins, having passed from the deep to the superficial veins through the communicating veins.

When skeletal muscles contract, they compress the intra- and intermuscular veins, expelling their blood into any venous conduit less affected by the extrinsic pressure caused by the contraction. Venous valves prevent retrograde flow and ensure that emptied segments refill from the periphery during muscle relaxation.

As the muscles relax, blood drains rapidly from the distal veins into the emptied muscle veins. Distal venous pressure therefore falls. At the same time, the proximal valves close and interrupt the vertical column of blood between limb and heart. This decreases venous pressure in the foot and calf from around 90–100 mm Hg in the immobile upright position to 20 mm Hg during walking, running and cycling. Reduced distal venous pressure increases the arteriovenous pressure difference driving blood flow through the calf muscle by 50–60%. With exercise, pressures in the normal saphenous vein (at the level of the malleolae) and posterior tibial vein fall 40–68 mm Hg below the resting level.

The peripheral venous pump consists of a number of separate but functionally integrated components. Each minor fascial compartment acts as a muscle pump unit. These may be considered in regional groups, as follows:

- the plantar or foot pump
- the calf pump (including the anterior tibial and peroneal pump)
- the thigh pump
- the abdominal pump.

Foot Pump

A venous foot pump was first postulated by le Dentu in 1867. The deep veins of the sole are connected with the superficial veins of the dorsum of the foot by communicating veins, which are either unvalved or have valves that allow flow from the deep to the superficial vein. Le Dentu and more recent authors concluded that the plantar venous pump empties blood from the deep to the superficial system by the direct pressure of weight-bearing and plantar muscle contraction. That this view is erroneous has been demonstrated by Doppler velocimetry and videophlebography.

The plantar venous pump consists essentially of the venae comitantes of the lateral plantar artery. The veins are slung like a bowstring and are emptied on weight-bearing by being stretched rather than by direct pressure. The contained blood does not empty into the superficial veins because the tension in the plantar aponeurosis closes the communicating veins. Therefore, the plantar venous pump empties primarily via the deep conduits of the calf.

It was thought previously that during walking, the deep venous foot pump could not empty into the deep veins of the calf because the muscles would be contracted. However, during the plantigrade weight-bearing phase of ambulation, the calf muscles are relaxed. They contract only later to facilitate heel lift. Furthermore, the deep veins of the calf are relatively protected from the pressures generated by contraction by virtue of the deep fascial sheath in which they are contained.

The LSV and SSV provide alternative channels for the venous drainage of the foot. The foot pump empties into these vessels if the calf muscles are contracted tightly, especially if the leg is warm and the superficial veins are dilated. The capacity of the plantar foot pump is in the region of 20 ml, and it is sufficiently powerful to dislocate a column of blood up to the heart.

Calf Pump

The calf pump has been called the "peripheral heart". The action of the calf pump is best understood if the superficial and deep veins are considered as two compartments with interconnections via the communicating veins. When the calf muscles contract, they raise the pressure in and around the structures contained within the deep fascia. All the intramuscular veins are emptied completely because the muscles generate extrinsic pressures of 200–300 mm Hg. The pressure surrounding the intermuscular veins does not rise as high, but it reaches levels of 100–150 mm Hg. These pressures empty the veins, the valves ensuring that blood flows towards the heart. Similarly, flow from the deep to the superficial compartment is prevented by the valves in the communicating veins. This has been demonstrated by serial phlebography of the normal lower leg.

The average volume of the calf is 1500–2000 ml, and the calf blood volume is 60–70 ml. Continuous exercise reduces the calf blood volume by 1.5–2 ml/100 ml, mostly by compression of the intramuscular veins. The average expelled volume is approximately 30–40 ml, i.e. 50% of all the blood within the calf. The calf pump can expel this volume in four to five contractions, although almost as much can be achieved by one single sustained contraction. With increased exercise, muscle blood flow may increase to 20–30 ml/100 ml/min, which places an additional load of 600 ml/min on the calf pump. The calf must contract at least 20 times every minute to expel this increased blood flow. Normal walking, at 80 steps a minute, contracts each calf 40 times a minute, so the pump can deal easily with the high blood flow of exercise hyperaemia.

The outflow conduit from the calf pump is a very large-bore vein with virtually no resistance to flow. Since the gradient of 10–15 mm Hg between the small veins and the heart is sufficient to ensure venous blood flow when the subject is supine, the increase in gradient to 100–200 mm Hg produced by the calf pump ensures rapid venous return to the heart during vigorous erect muscle exercise.

As the calf muscles start to relax, the deep veins are empty and therefore are unaffected by hydrostatic pressure. The superficial veins however are full and subject to hydrostatic pressure plus the vis a tergo remnant. The pressure gradient between the two compartments is therefore 100–110 mm Hg. Just as blood flows from the left atrium to the left ventricle during ventricular diastole, so blood flows from the superficial to the deep compartment when the calf muscles relax. The superficial compartment empties incompletely and its pressure falls. Superficial vein pressure during exercise falls by 60–80%, and this reduction is essential for the preservation of healthy skin and subcutaneous tissues.

It is important to realise that while contraction is the main activator of the venous pump, stretching a muscle also raises the intramuscular pressure and promotes emptying of the contained veins. This is particularly important in the foot pump. Pressures of 35 mm Hg have been recorded in the tibialis anterior during stretching, and the distal calf pump acts in similar fashion. Thus, peripheral muscle pump activity performs four vital functions:

- It ensures rapid adequate venous return from the lower limbs during exercise to replenish a falling CVP.
- It reduces superficial vein pressure, thus removing the potentially damaging effect of the hydrostatic pressure that is inseparable from man's upright posture.
- Since capillary pressure is closer to venous than to arterial pressure, the muscle pump reduces capillary filtration in the legs.
- It increases lymph flow by intermittent compression of lymph vessels. Exercise therefore reduces the tendency of the dependant limb to swell.

Thigh Pump

Each of the three muscle groups in the thigh, with its enveloping fascia and contained veins, acts as a pumping unit. It is probable that the transfer of blood from the superficial to the deep veins, and towards the heart, is achieved by a mechanism similar to that in the calf. The sartorius muscle is uniquely placed to compress the femoral vein and may act as an additional muscle pump in the thigh.

Abdominal Pump

Inspiration increases intra-abdominal pressure. The pressures in the external and common iliac veins and inferior vena cava therefore rise by 6.3 mm Hg and 8.7 mm Hg in the horizontal and erect positions, respectively. This demonstrates the existence of an abdominal component of the peripheral venous pump, which is greater when the subject is erect.

Movements of the diaphragm affect the resistance of the outflow conduit because they change abdominal and thoracic pressure. During inspiration, abdominal pressure increases, and this decreases venous return from the lower limb. The decreasing thoracic pressure increases the pressure gradient between the abdomen and the thorax, encouraging venous blood flow from the abdominal to the thoracic veins. Thus, during inspiration, blood flow from the limbs to the abdomen is impeded, but blood flow from the abdomen to the thorax is accelerated. However, deep inspiration results in a paradoxical resistance phenomenon caused by the diaphragm exerting a squeezing action on the inferior vena cava. Blood flow drops from 20 ml/s to near-zero and cardiac oscillations are no longer visible in the caval pressure.

With quiet expiration, the abdominal pressure falls and venous blood flow recommences from the lower limbs to the abdomen. A positive but smaller pressure gradient between the abdomen and chest maintains blood flow from the abdomen to the chest. Forced expiration, coughing or a Valsalva manoeuvre can elevate intrathoracic pressure to 400 mm Hg, and paroxysmal coughing can impede venous inflow to such a degree that fainting results.

Conclusion

Our understanding of venous physiology of the lower limbs has increased dramatically in the past decade. That gravity increases pressure in the veins of the lower limb during orthostasis and contributes to the development of varicose veins in man is undisputed. However, the numerous studies of venous pressure in the dependent limb neglect the fact that the physiological response to increased pressure in a normal vein is hypertrophy, not dilation. This is demonstrated in the medial muscular hypertrophy seen in reversed saphenous vein used as arterial bypass grafts. Equating pressure to flow is a cardinal error that has led previously to erroneous assumptions that blood flow in the foot is from deep to superficial veins and that venous return in the dependent limb must first overcome gravity.

Turbulence causes a greatly increased shear force on the endothelium and was suggested as a possible major factor in the development of superficial varices as early as 1972. Eight years later, it was discovered that endothelial release of EDRF (nitric oxide) results in local vasodilation. It is now known that altered shear forces stimulate nitric oxide production. A dynamic concept of perturbations in flow rather than a static picture of chronically elevated venous pressure therefore appears more likely as the *sine qua non* in the aetiology of varicose veins.

4

Investigations of the Lower-limb Venous System

S. Sarin

Early tests of venous function all relied on clinical examination of the affected limb. Fabry in 1589 is credited with first describing "instantaneous" descent of blood into the veins of a raised leg made dependent in a patient with a leg ulcer. In 1846, Brodie formalised this observation by describing his test of venous valvular function where, after having emptied the veins of the leg, he demonstrated that the reflux could be controlled by pressure on the vein above. The test was popularised by Trendelenburg in the 1890s and is now standard clinical practice. The first description of a test to assess muscle pump function was by Perthes in 1895. The superficial veins were constricted proximally and the patient was made to walk. The superficial varicosities would disappear only if the valves of the deep system were competent. With some minor modifications, these tests remain the standard clinical investigations of venous function. With the development of sophisticated, objective, non-invasive tests, the value of the clinical tests of venous function is being called into question. Clinical tests are subjective, hence prone to observer-dependent error, and they are unsuitable for all but the simplest assessment of venous function, e.g. whether there is any evidence of venous disease, or whether it is the long or short saphenous system that is affected. The ultimate purpose of any test of venous function is to make a diagnosis that will direct treatment. The test, or combination of tests, must be able to assess the competence of the deep venous system, identify superficial venous disease, and locate the source of retrograde flow. Modern tests can be split broadly into those that look at venous morphology and direction of flow and those that assess overall venous function. Both types of test have their place and are used commonly to complement the information derived from clinical examination.

Venous Morphology and Direction of Blood Flow

Doppler

The principle that the frequency of a wave reflected from a moving object is changed in proportion to the velocity of the reflecting object is the basis of Doppler flow detection. Handheld ultrasound Doppler probes have been in widespread use for many years. Venous reflux testing may be performed with the patient standing in a modification of the Trendelenburg test. The femoral vein and saphenofemoral junction can be examined by insonating with the Doppler probe and locating the femoral vein lying medial to the femoral artery. Calf compression is applied by the examiner's hand or by a rapidly inflating cuff to produce forward flow, which may be detected in the groin. On relaxation of calf compression, a search is made for venous reflux. This is seen easily as an upward deflection of the trace when using a bidirectional Doppler system in connection with a chart recorder, or its characteristic sound can be sought without such complexity. The popliteal fossa can be examined similarly, searching for popliteal vein or SSV reflux. Narrow cuffs or tourniquets can be used to compress the superficial veins and assist in the differentiation of superficial from deep venous reflux. This method has the inherent difficulty that it is qualitative; more importantly, it is difficult to determine which vein is being examined, particularly in the popliteal fossa.

Duplex Scanning

The combination of Doppler ultrasound with real-time B-mode imaging has provided a means for the localisation of the Doppler sample volume on the ultrasound image. The pulsed Doppler mode means that precisely defined areas can be studied to determine the velocity and direction of flow. The presence of flow in major vessels can be established and the location of venous reflux determined beyond doubt. The lower-limb vessels may be identified in turn, with the patient standing or lying with the feet dependent. Forward flow can be produced in the calf by manual calf compression, and the presence of forward flow and reflux can be assessed in each vein of the lower limb in turn. Virtually all veins below the inguinal ligament can be imaged by this technique, and the competence of individual valves can be determined. It has been shown to have a good correlation with venography in the assessment of venous reflux and thrombosis.

Colour-flow mapping of the Doppler signal provides additional sophistication. The Doppler shift of each pixel of the ultrasound image is converted to a colour of different saturation depending on the velocity of flow. In effect, real-time images with colours representing the flow of blood (e.g. blue for blood flowing away from the probe, red for blood flowing towards the probe) are obtained, which simplifies assessment of venous reflux. Other advantages of duplex scanning are that it is entirely non-invasive and can be repeated easily with minimum discomfort to the subject. The main disadvantage of duplex scanning in the assessment of venous disorders is that it is operator-dependent. Firstly, if the test is undertaken by a technician inexperienced in the surgical management of venous disease, then interpretation of the results can be difficult. Secondly, the accuracy of the test diminishes as one looks at the calf veins (either for reflux or thrombosis). Keeping these two points in mind, this test is extremely useful in the assessment of primary varicose veins, recurrent varicose veins, preoperative marking of the saphenopopliteal junction, venous assessment of lower-limb ulcers, and diagnosis of DVT. Figures 4.1–4.5 show examples of duplex images obtained in various venous conditions.

Venography

Venography was the first means of investigating the venous system and is still in wide use today. Use of this modality enables direct assessment of the superficial and deep venous systems and an evaluation of venous valvular function. In experienced hands, images of lower-limb veins can be obtained, and it is still regarded by many as a reference standard in the investigation of DVT. Modifications (retrograde/

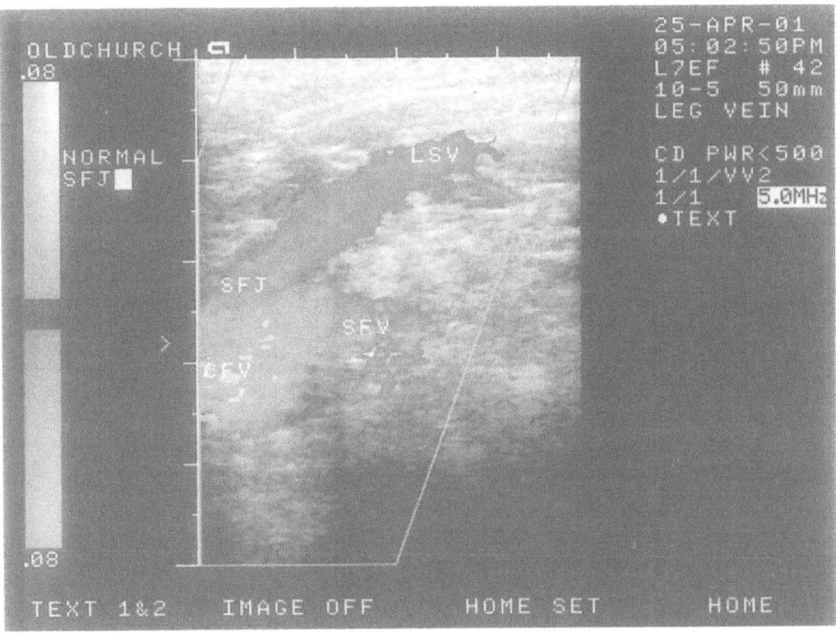

Figure 4.1 Normal saphenofemoral junction (SFJ), long saphenous vein (LSV), superficial femoral vein (SFV), and common femoral vein (CFV). Also Plate I.

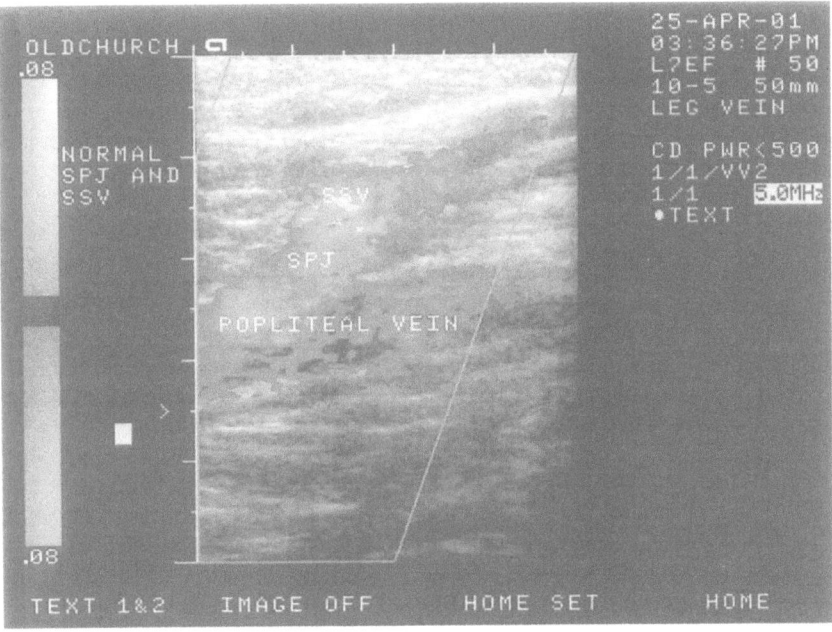

Figure 4.2 Normal saphenopopliteal junction (SPJ), short saphenous vein (SSV), and popliteal vein. Also Plate I.

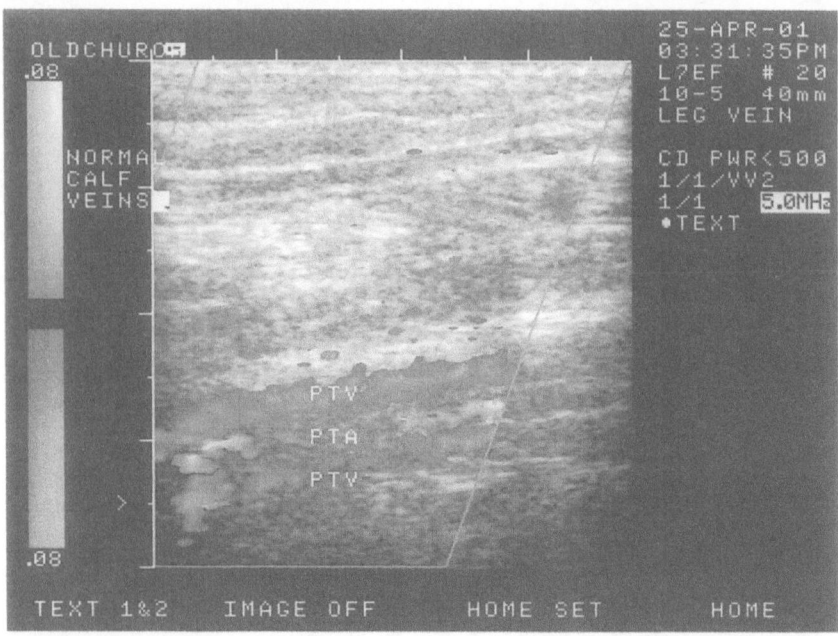

Figure 4.3 Normal posterior tibial artery (PTA) and paired posterior tibial veins (PTV). Also Plate II.

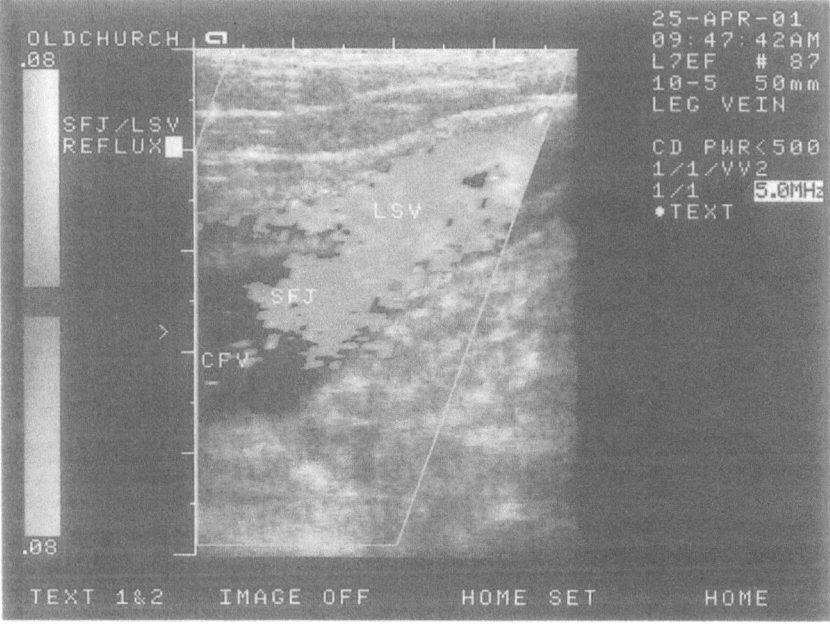

Figure 4.4 Reflux (red is set as reverse flow) in saphenofemoral junction (SFJ) and long saphenous vein (SFV). Also Plate II.

CFV, common femoral vein.

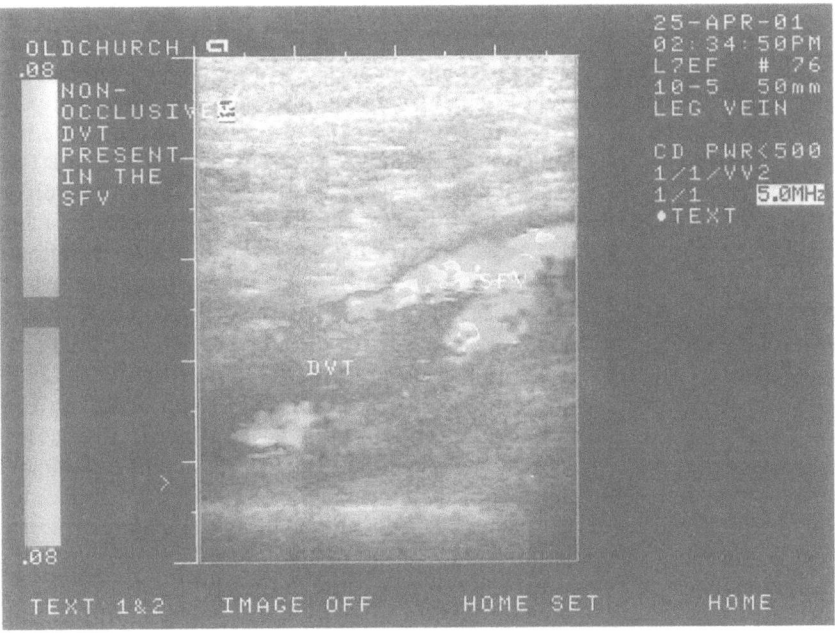

Figure 4.5 Deep venous thrombosis (DVT; appears as filling defect) in superficial femoral vein (SFV). Also Plate III.

descending venography) to permit the assessment of valve competence in the deep and superficial systems have been described. In clinical practice, ascending venography is used to detect evidence of venous thrombosis; descending venography is used to detect evidence of venous reflux. Varicography also has a place in the assessment of pelvic varices and is sometimes used intraoperatively to locate the saphenopopliteal junction.

However, venography necessitates expensive equipment (the use of real-time screening is highly desirable), is uncomfortable for patients, and exposes patients to ionising radiation. Repeated radiological studies to assess the progression of venous disease are clearly undesirable. With the advent of duplex scanning, many practitioners have found venography to be of little value in general clinical practice, although some still use it to assess patients before deep venous reconstructive procedures.

Evaluation of Venous Function

Ambulatory Venous Pressure

Ambulatory venous pressure (AVP) measurement has been proposed as the gold standard for the assessment of venous function. Since the original measurements by Pollack and Wood in the late 1940s, it has been recognised that a persistently raised superficial dorsal foot vein pressure during exercise is associated with venous disease.

Originally, a dorsal foot vein was cannulated and a catheter connected to a water manometer. More recently, this has been modified by the use of a pressure transducer, which can be used to convert the pressure to an electrical signal that can be recorded by a chart recorder or computer. Using commonly available equipment, it is possible to investigate functional abnormalities of the lower-limb venous system. The test is very simple: after cannulation of the dorsal foot vein, the patient undertakes a standard exercise to test the calf muscle pump. The patient walks on a treadmill until a stable pressure is reached, usually within 10–20 seconds. The pressure reached at the end of exercise is the AVP. The venous system then refills from arterial inflow and venous reflux, if present. The time taken to return to the pre-exercise pressure is the venous refilling time. Various indices have been described that combine these two aspects of the refilling curve to give a single figure of venous function. Under normal circumstances, venous pressure should fall to less than 20 mm Hg during exercise and return to normal over a period of not less than 20 seconds. This test can be repeated using tourniquets or narrow cuffs to occlude the superficial veins of the thigh and leg in order to permit an assessment of the contribution of superficial and deep venous reflux to the physiological abnormality observed, in a manner similar to that used in the Trendelenburg test. This technique permits the objective investigation of the venous muscle pump function in the whole leg, but it does not give precise anatomical information regarding the cause of the problem.

Plethysmography

Plethysmography includes a number of tests that detect volume changes in a limb, which give an indication of limb or regional blood flow and, hence, an index of degree of functional incompetence. Methods used include the use of strain gauges applied to segments of the limb (strain-gauge plethysmography), airbag sleeves (air plethysmography), and the assessment of differential haemoglobin absorption (photoplethysmography, PPG).

Air Plethysmography

This test is based on volume changes detected by an air-containing compartment or cuff wrapped around part or all of the calf. The cuff is inflated with air to a low pressure, so that fluctuations of calf volume are reflected by a change of pressure within the cuff. The technique has been known for many years, but recently modern materials have permitted simplification of the equipment. The first descriptions of the equipment, using pneumatic cuffs inflated around short sections of the leg, employed various manoeuvres to assess venous function. These included quickly tilting the patient from head-up to head-down to assess the rate of venous outflow in the diagnosis of DVT. The reverse manoeuvre was used to measure venous reflux.

In the modern version, a plastic sleeve is zipped around the patient's leg and filled with air to a pressure of 6–8 mm Hg. This is sufficient to ensure close conformity with the leg but does not interfere with the venous physiology under study. It is now possible for the device to be calibrated so absolute volume changes in the limb can be measured. The patient undertakes a series of exercises, standing on their toes once and then ten times. The ejected volume after one and then ten tiptoe exercises can be calculated, as can the venous refilling time following exercise. This allows a full assessment of the calf muscle pump to be undertaken, as well as an estimate of the contribution of superficial venous reflux by the application of narrow cuffs or tourniquets. Substantial cooperation from the patient is required, since they must stand on both feet during the exercise phase and then on only one foot during the recovery period. Thermal drift of the plethysmograph may be encountered as the patient's warmth heats the air within the cuff, causing an increase in pressure.

Strain-gauge Plethysmography

This method has been used for several years in the assessment of patients with venous disease and is employed to quantify the changes in volume of the calf that occur during exercise or compression of the limb with cuffs. Originally made of mercury in a rubber tube, the transducer is now made from a mercury-filled silastic tube. This is stretched around the calf, ankle or foot. The electrical resistance of the tube is dependent on the length and related inversely to the cross-sectional area of the mercury column. As the calf increases in volume, the silastic tube stretches, increasing in length but decreasing in cross-section. This results in an increase in the resistance of the mercury column. The advantage of this system is that the changes in resistance relate directly to changes in volume, permitting satisfactory volumetric calibration of the strain-gauge system.

Mercury-in-silastic strain-gauge plethysmography was originally designed to measure venous outflow from the limb to quantify proximal venous obstruction. Later, it was adapted to measure the severity of venous reflux. This was done with the leg supine and the strain gauge applied around the calf. A proximal thigh cuff inflated to 250–300 mm Hg was used to occlude arterial inflow; then the distal thigh cuffs were inflated rapidly to 50 mm Hg. Venous blood beneath the distal cuff was displaced distally by this method, and the change in volume of the calf was measured by the strain-gauge plethysmograph.

This technique was subsequently adapted to be performed with the patient standing while undertaking tiptoe exercises or walking on a treadmill. Arterial occlusion cuffs are not employed in this position; instead, tourniquets are used to differentiate between deep and superficial vein incompetence, in a similar fashion to the other venous reflux tests. The technique has been validated against both venography and venous-pressure measurements. However, only the small area of the limb beneath the strain gauge is measured, and slippage of the gauge is a potential source of error. Mercury is potentially toxic and tends to oxidise after about one year's use, resulting in failure of the gauge. This has been overcome by the introduction of an indium–gallium alloy, which is less prone to these difficulties. The main value of this test is in the identification of the small number of patients in whom the main problem is one of venous obstruction.

Photoplethysmography

PPG uses variation in light absorption in the skin to estimate indirectly changes in venous volume. The principal chromophore in the skin is haemoglobin, so light absorption is dependent largely on the volume of blood in the superficial dermal venous plexuses. When these are full, the haemoglobin in the red blood cells absorbs light; as venous pressure falls, the plexuses become emptier and light absorption decreases. The method uses an infrared (805 nm) light-emitting diode within a probe fixed to the skin by double-sided adhesive tape, and a photoelectric cell arranged within the probe so that it measures light reflected from the skin. Following a standard procedure to empty the veins (e.g. repeated dorsiflexion of the ankle in a sitting patient), a graph reflecting the changes in light backscatter is obtained. This represents the emptying of the limb during muscle contraction followed by gradual refilling during relaxation. It reflects both the action of the muscle pump in emptying the dermal venous plexus and the presence of reflux within the superficial or deep venous systems allowing rapid venous refilling. From the trace, various indices can be measured, including the venous emptying and refilling times. The total refilling time, 95% refilling time (as the upward slope may level off slightly or overshoot before returning to the baseline), 50% refilling time (t1/2), and the gradient of the slope have been suggested as standard measurements. A 95% refilling time is used by most laboratories, and a value of less than 20 seconds has been regarded as evidence of venous reflux, although individual laboratories have to calculate their own values. The test is of little value in the primary diagnosis of venous disease. The author reserves it to assess, in the presence of deep venous insufficiency, the contribution of coexistent superficial venous disease to overall venous function.

Conclusion

In the setting of a modern vascular clinic, clinical examination and selective use of the above tests are desirable to ensure a pathophysiological diagnosis that will define the correct treatment options for the patient. For example, in young patients suspected of having primary varicose veins in the distribution of the long saphenous system, clinical examination supplemented by handheld Doppler usually suffices. In patients with varicosities in the short saphenous system or with recurrent varicose veins, clinical examination and Duplex scanning are essential to locate precisely the source of reflux and to rule out deep venous insufficiency. Patients with more complex venous disease may require air or strain-gauge plethysmography, PPG, venography, or a combination of these in addition to Duplex scanning.

5 Compression Treatment for Venous Disease of the Lower Limb

A. Abu-Own

Compression bandages were used for the treatment of leg ulcers by the ancient Egyptians. Hippocrates advocated the use of compression in the treatment of venous disease. Celsus used plasters and linen bandages for ulcers, and Ibn-Sina (also known as Avicenna) used wine-soaked compresses. Henri de Mondeville also recognised that compression bandaging helped heal ulcers, but, like Hippocrates and Ibn-Sina, claimed that they did so by driving out "evil humours".

Wiseman's leather lace-up stocking may be regarded as the first graduated compression design; the use of such an ingenious design meant that the desired level of compression could be maintained after the leg swelling was reduced. Wiseman emphasised the importance of varicose veins in the development of leg ulcers and introduced the term "varicose ulcer".

Spender in 1866 stressed that bandages should be applied properly and "when possible, be executed by the surgeon in attendance". Dickson Wright in 1930 and Bisgaard in 1948 described the use of elastic bandages. The advent of elastic fibres led to the development of the modern elastic stockings.

Graduated Compression

Theoretical considerations and physiological measurements suggest that leg compression should be graduated, being maximal at the gaiter area and diminishing proximally. Van der Molen in 1982 introduced the idea of graduated compression. Sigg suggested that the greatest pressure should be applied over the gaiter (ulcer-bearing) area. A number of calf-pump function studies have shown improved venous return with graduated stockings. The compression applied should be approximately 75% at the upper calf and 50% at the thigh compared with the compression applied at the ankle.

Types of Compression

Compression is usually applied continuously to the leg as graduated static compression using stockings or bandages. Alternatively, intermittent pneumatic compression (IPC) may be used.

Bandages

Bandages are preferred following sclerotherapy and venous surgery and for open leg ulcers, particularly where soiling through dressings is frequent. Bandages are relatively cheap and, with appropriate training, easy to apply. The main advantage over stockings, however, is that bandages can accommodate any size and shape of leg. One frequently encounters patients with legs that off-the-shelf stockings would not fit; a stocking that is not a proper fit will fail to produce the desired effects and occasionally can do harm. Attention to detail in the application of bandages is of paramount importance. An overlapping figure-of-eight technique is more effective than a simple spiral bandage for achieving and sustaining the desirable level of compression. The importance of graduated compression has been mentioned above and applies to both bandages and stockings.

Single-layer bandages maintain pressure poorly, and the pressure under the bandage may decrease to inadequate levels within a few hours. The favourable results achieved by the Charing Cross method are attributed to the application of a four-layer bandaging technique, involving wool (absorbent), crepe, elastic bandage (e.g. Elset by Seton), and adhesive bandage (e.g. Coban from 3M). Ulcer healing rates of up to 75% at 12 weeks have been achieved using this technique.

Stockings

For the majority of patients with venous disease, compression stockings are more appropriate than bandages. Once ulcer healing is achieved using bandages, it is important to continue leg compression using stockings to reduce the risk of ulcer recurrence. This should be stressed to both the primary healthcare personnel and the patients.

Many types of compression stockings are available, but only a few conform to acceptable standards. A unit interested in the management of venous disease should check the manufacturers' specifications regarding pressures and gradients claimed for their stockings. Cornwall and colleagues studied 15 types of below-knee compression garments; only five of these met certain criteria, which included satisfactory graduation. When tested on patients with chronic venous insufficiency (CVI), the five garments with satisfactory graduation improved PPG refilling time significantly, while those with unsatisfactory graduation had less effect.

Classes of Compression Stockings

Manufacturers use wooden legs and fabric-testing machines to test their leg-compression products (indirect measurements). However, pressures specified by the manufacturers on the basis of such indirect laboratory tests do not usually reflect the actual pressures measured on patients. Direct methods (in situ pressure measurements) are clinically more relevant. The Borgnis medical stocking tester (MST) is used to measure pressure directly from underneath bandages or stockings and is the most popular of the direct methods.

Medical stockings are usually classified into four classes on the basis of the pressure produced at the ankle. Table 5.1 summarises the uses of each class.

A higher compression is likely to improve calf pump function to a greater degree and to achieve better clinical results. However, in practice, for many patients a lower compression class may be prescribed to achieve better compliance, e.g. class II com-

Table 5.1 Graduated compression classes and their recommended uses

Class	Pressure at ankle (mm Hg)	Indications
I	18–25	DVT prophylaxis, varicose veins
II	25–35	DVT prophylaxis in pregnancy, sclerotherapy, marked varicose veins, venous surgery, superficial thrombophlebitis
III	35–45	CVI, lymphoedema
IV	45–60	Severe CVI with oedema, lymphoedema

pression is often prescribed for many patients with CVI. For long-term use of stockings, it is common practice to prescribe two pairs of stockings every six months.

Intermittent Pneumatic Compression

IPC may be used as an alternative or in addition to static compression in the prophylaxis of DVT. IPC may be applied to the calf using a single-chamber device or through a series of chambers inflated sequentially from the ankle to the thigh. In a recent study, the use of the sequential compression device has been shown to enhance venous ulcer healing.

IPC may be applied to the foot, utilising the venous foot pump and producing haemodynamic effects similar to those produced by walking. This method has been shown to be effective in reducing post-traumatic swelling and in the prevention of DVT.

Elastic or Non-elastic Compression?

The advent of elastic fibre, which led to the manufacture of elastic stockings and bandages, was without doubt a major advance in compression therapy. Elastic bandages maintained pressure more effectively and have been shown to achieve better rates of ulcer healing. However, non-elastic compression exerts less pressure when the patient is lying, making them safer in patients with arterial impairment and diabetics.

Below-knee or Thigh-length Compression?

For the majority of patients with CVI, knee-length stockings or bandages are appropriate. This is sufficient to assist the calf muscle pump as well as allowing a possible enhancement of the skin microcirculation in the gaiter area. Short stockings are easier to put on, and compliance with them is better. Occasionally, thigh-length stockings may be indicated because limb swelling is extending into the thigh or on account of the patient's preference. In DVT prophylaxis, a thigh-length stocking is normally used.

Indications for Compression Treatment in Venous Disease

Varicose Veins

Support stockings are often prescribed for patients with varicose veins as a method of relieving symptoms. Stockings for patients with varicose veins are prescribed either as a definitive treatment or temporarily for those awaiting surgery. There is considerable debate as to how external support produces symptomatic relief in patients with varicose veins. Somerville and colleagues evaluated the effect of elastic stockings on ambulatory venous pressure in 12 patients and suggested that external elastic support may produce a reduction in ambulatory venous pressure. More recent studies, however, have failed to confirm this. One recent study evaluated the continuing use of stockings following varicose vein surgery. It showed reduced recurrence in the stockings group, but compliance was poor. Further work is required to assess these findings.

Varicose Vein Surgery

Firm leg compression is usually applied following varicose vein surgery. At the end of the operation, such compression helps to stop bleeding and to reduce postoperative bruising. It also reduces oedema and may reduce the risk of DVT. Elastocrepe bandage is usually applied initially; this can be changed subsequently to elastic compression stocking.

Superficial Thrombophlebitis

Once superficial thrombophlebitis has developed, it is usually treated conservatively by external compression and anti-inflammatory analgesics until the acute inflammatory condition has subsided. If the underlying cause is varicose veins, then appropriate elective surgery may be performed to prevent further attacks. Acute surgical treatment by flush ligation with and without removal of the entire phlebitic vein has been advocated by some authors.

In the short term, thrombophlebitis of a varicose vein may appear to achieve the same effect as compression sclerotherapy. However, most of these veins recanalise because they are full of thrombus. A varicose vein treated properly by compression sclerotherapy should be free of thrombus and is less likely to recanalise.

Compression Sclerotherapy

Foote referred to a number of clinicians who have attempted, since the middle of the nineteenth century, to obliterate varicose veins by injecting them with a variety of solutions. Linser in 1916 was, however, the first to describe the use of compression bandages after the injection of sclerosant. He used hypertonic saline, which caused considerable pain and often resulted in skin necrosis. A number of safer sclerosants have been developed since. Sodium tetradecyl sulphate was developed by Tournay in Paris in the 1930s and is still the most commonly used sclerosant today.

The technique, described in Chapter 7, involves injection of the sclerosant into an almost empty vein followed by immediate application of compression. This ensures the development of a controlled sterile phlebitis with a minimal-diameter thrombus within the collapsed vein. Compression maintains lumen occlusion by making opposing surfaces stick together with minimal intervening thrombus. The vein is permanently obliterated and replaced by a thin fibrosed (sclerosed) cord incapable of recanalisation. Compression is provided by using foam rubber pads and bandaging the leg.

Chronic Venous Insufficiency and Venous Ulceration

Most patients with CVI, with or without venous ulceration, benefit from compression therapy. For many patients with CVI, leg compression remains the mainstay of their treatment; the majority of these are patients with post-thrombotic deep venous insufficiency who, at present, cannot be cured by surgery.

Compression Stockings and Chronic Swelling of the Leg

Patients are often referred for assessment in a vascular laboratory because of leg swelling. The common systemic causes of leg swelling, such as cardiac failure, renal failure and hypoproteinaemia, should normally be excluded before such a referral. The local causes of leg swelling may be inflammatory, lymphatic or venous.

Leg swelling in venous disease is caused by chronic venous hypertension, causing an increase in capillary pressure and disturbing the Starling's equilibrium for capillary exchange. Treatment of oedema in venous disease should, if possible, be directed at correcting the cause of venous hypertension. However, in severe oedema, general measures such as limb elevation, physiotherapy, and leg compression, should be considered as part of the management regimen. In the treatment of venous ulceration associated with severe local oedema, Ruckley (1992; see *Further Reading*) recommends that patients be admitted to hospital for bedrest with leg elevation, followed by compression treatment and mobilisation.

Deep Vein Thrombosis Prophylaxis

Graduated compression stockings have been shown to be effective and are used widely in the prevention of DVT and pulmonary embolism. Stockings should be applied immediately following admission to hospital to prevent preoperative thrombosis. The risk of postoperative thromboembolic disease continues for several weeks after discharge from hospital. Further studies are required to investigate the effectiveness and duration of post-discharge thromboprophylaxis.

Modern stockings are comfortable to wear and can be used for DVT prophylaxis in most types of patients without adverse effects. Compression stockings for DVT prophylaxis are graduated, producing 20 mm Hg compression at the ankle. The minimal compression of these stockings in the thigh and the careful design of their tops help to prevent a tendency to a tourniquet effect around the thighs.

Graduated compression stockings are also used as an adjunct to other therapy in the treatment of DVT. Once anticoagulant therapy is established and firm compression applied, patients may be encouraged to mobilise without causing a higher risk of pulmonary embolism. A report by Partsch suggested that even patients with pelvic vein thrombosis could be treated with firm compression and anticoagulation without immobilisation.

IPC has also been used widely in the prophylaxis of DVT. Several studies have shown that the incidence of DVT is reduced by the perioperative application of IPC to the lower limb. In a compilation of 11 studies on 902 general surgical patients, IPC reduced the incidence of DVT from 20% to 9.6%. This method can be used either alone or in conjunction with another mechanical or pharmacological method of thromboprophylaxis. Its use in combination with graduated compression stockings has been demonstrated to be superior to using either of the two methods alone. In a case meta-analysis, the incidence of DVT was reduced from an average of 27% in controls to 4.5% in patients who received stockings plus IPC prophylaxis. It is simple to use and free of the haemorrhagic complications that may be associated with pharmacological methods. It is thought that IPC increases blood flow velocity in the deep veins, thereby counteracting venous stasis, one of Virchow's triad of the causes of thrombosis. The suggestion that IPC stimulates the release of fibrinolytic activator from the endothelium has not been confirmed in a recent study.

IPC may be applied either as uniform compression to the calf using a single-chamber device, or through a series of chambers inflated in a sequential manner from ankle to thigh to achieve venous emptying. The latter method was designed for use in the prevention of DVT and has been investigated in many studies, which have confirmed its efficacy. A study by Abu-Own, Scurr and Coleridge Smith (1993; see *Further Reading*) suggested that sequential intermittent pneumatic compression of the calf and thigh (using a sequential compression device manufactured by Kendall) is less likely to cause distal blood trapping and foot swelling than single-chamber calf compression. Other commonly used mechanical methods for DVT prophylaxis include the Flowtron boot and Footpump; the former is also used in the treatment of lymphoedema.

Effectiveness of Compression Therapy

There is no doubt that compression therapy is effective in venous disease. It heals ulcers and keeps them healed if compression treatment is maintained. For many patients with CVI and venous ulceration, long-term leg compression remains the mainstay of their management. When compression therapy fails, it is often an indication to check that an appropriate type of compression has been applied correctly and to assess the patient's compliance. It is also generally accepted that graduated elastic compression and IPC are effective in DVT prophylaxis.

How does Compression Treatment Work?

Despite the widespread agreement on its efficacy, the mechanism by which compression treatment works remains largely unknown. Decreased fibrinolytic activity in blood and tissues has been reported in patients with venous disease. It has been suggested that external compression may encourage the release of fibrinolytic activators from the venous endothelium and improve tissue fibrinolysis. Burnand in 1980 reported that fibrinolytic enhancement and elastic stockings reduced oedema and improved calf pump function.

Recently, the controversy has been mainly about the aspects of venous function that are influenced by compression. Previous studies have focused attention on studying the effects of compression on the overall venous haemodynamics of the lower limb. In patients with CVI, the ambulatory foot vein pressure is raised, and it might be hoped that compression stockings would restore this index to normal. Some authors have found that this is the case, but others have failed to find any effect. The time required for the foot vein pressure to return to resting levels after the end of exercise is an indicator of the degree of reflux in a limb. Whether measured by air plethysmography, strain-gauge plethysmography, foot volumetry, or foot vein pressures, variable results have been obtained, with only some authors reporting a

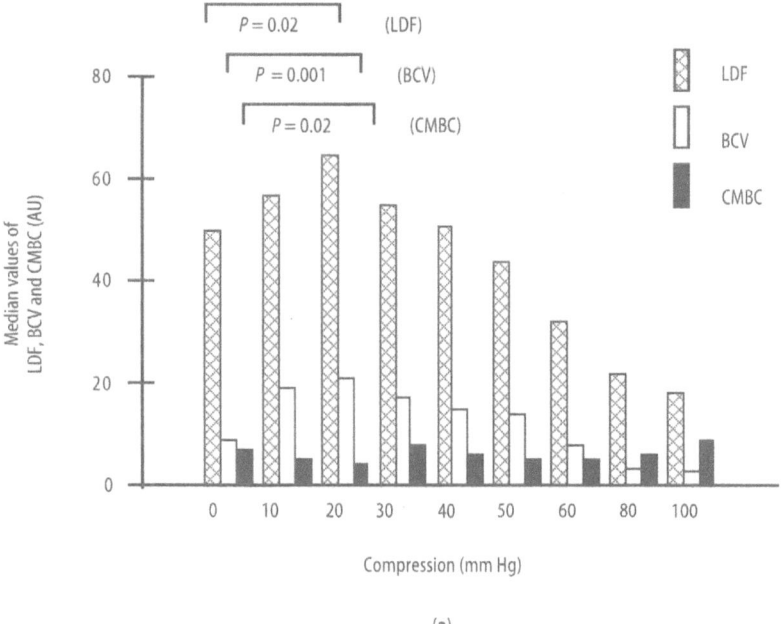

(a)

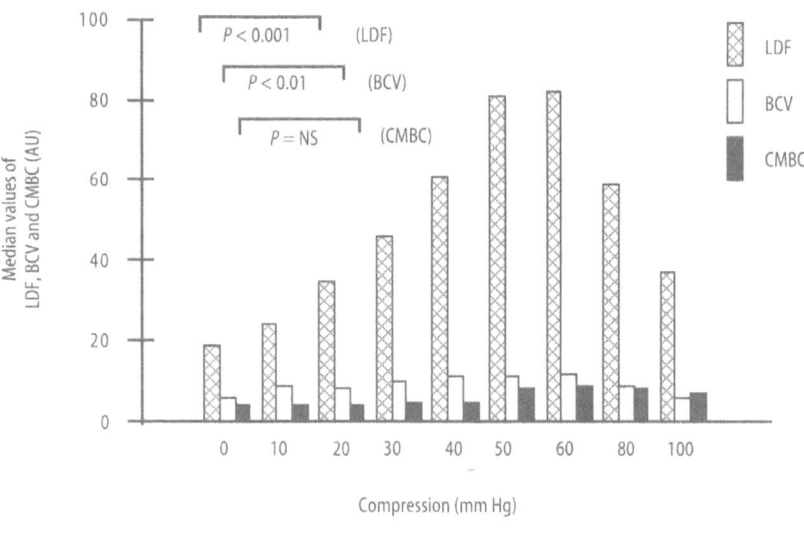

(b)

Figure 5.1 Effect of leg compression on laser Doppler flux (LDF), blood-cell velocity (BCV), and concentration of moving blood cells (CMBC) in patients with lipodermatosclerosis. (a) Horizontal position; (b) dependent position. The medians of LDF, BCV and CMBC are plotted in arbitrary units (AU).

NS, not significant; *P*, Wilcoxon matched-pairs signed-ranks test comparing the values at 20 mm Hg compression with the basal values at 0 mm Hg.

beneficial effect. Air plethysmography may permit a more detailed analysis of the calf muscle pump, yet this has not demonstrated reduced venous refilling times after the application of stockings.

The effect of compressing incompetent popliteal veins, LSVs and SSVs while monitoring the presence of reflux using colour duplex ultrasound imaging has been studied recently. It was found that in the majority of veins, competence could not be restored without occluding the vein. In those patients where competence was restored before occlusion, much higher pressures were required than those exerted by conventional hosiery or bandages.

Abu-Own and colleagues (1994; see *Further Reading*) studied the effects of leg compression on the skin microcirculation. An experimental system was used to measure the effects of different degrees of compression on the microcirculatory blood flow in patients with lipodermatosclerosis. At 20 mm Hg compression in the supine position, there was a 33% median increase in laser Doppler flux, with a corresponding 79% median increase in blood cell velocity. It is interesting to note that the increase in laser Doppler flux with compression was attributable to an increase in blood-cell velocity, with no substantial alteration in the volume (concentration) of moving blood cells (Figure 5.1). In the dependent position, pressures up to 60 mm Hg caused an increase in laser Doppler flux and blood-cell velocity. In a further study, direct laser Doppler measurements from underneath a grade II compression stocking were made. The results were similar to those produced by the application of 20–30 mm Hg compression in the experimental model for leg compression.

It seems probable that stockings and compression bandaging may benefit the overall haemodynamics of the limb. However, this may play only a small part in the mechanism of action of compression. Leg compression results in significant alteration in the local microcirculatory blood flow; most obvious is an increase in blood-cell velocity in response to compression. Such an increase in velocity may reduce the likelihood of white blood cells in capillaries and venules interacting with the endothelium. Since it is possible that white blood cells play a significant role in the pathogenesis of venous disease, this suggests that compression stockings may be effective in the treatment of CVI by enhancing the microcirculatory flow velocity and preventing white-cell activation.

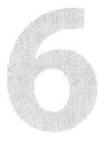

Histology of Veins and Thrombosis

G. Fegan and I. Saeed

Normal veins differ from arteries of the same size. The wall of a vein is thinner, and the three tunicae (intima, media, adventitia) are less well demarcated. The elastic tissue is scanty and not organised clearly into distinct internal and external elastic layers, and the medial smooth-muscle cells are relatively fewer in number, are separated widely by collagen fibres, and are arranged in circular and longitudinal fashions. All veins except the venae cavae and common iliac veins have valves. These valves, which are best developed in the leg veins, are paired folds of intimal tissue with collagen and elastin but little smooth muscle.

The principal age changes in veins are the development of a definite fibromuscular intimal layer, which is often eccentric in thickness at a given site. This intimal fibromuscular layer hyalinises with age and may calcify focally.

Varicose Veins

Histological changes in varicose veins are similar to, but more pronounced than, those of normal ageing. Calcification related to degeneration of medial elastic fibres may be present. Thrombosis is common, and organisation of the thrombi may lead to intimal fibrous and hyaline plaques.

Venous hypertension activates endothelial cells. These cells release inflammatory mediators and become adhesive for neutrophils, which are then activated. These activated leucocytes release free radicals and proteases, which are able to degrade the extracellular matrix. In addition hypoxia-activated endothelial cells secrete growth factors, which will trigger smooth-muscle cell proliferation and the synthesis of extracellular matrix.

Recanalisation of a Venous Thrombus

The object of all forms of sclerotherapy should be the production of a permanent fibrous occlusion of a vein at a point that will control retrograde pressure and flow. Such an occlusion develops over a period of time as a result of organisation of a thrombus produced deliberately. Three of the major pitfalls of this procedure are the production of uncontrolled thrombophlebitis and subsequent damage to normal valves; the formation of an occluding thrombus at a site that does not control the reflux of the superficial system; and the eventual recanalisation of the thrombus, which will result in the recurrence of symptoms.

The method of diagnosing and occluding the appropriate segment of vein is described in Chapter 7. This chapter is concerned with a description of the processes of thrombus organisation, and the way in which recanalisation can be prevented.

Hojensgard and Sturup in 1952 concluded from their investigations of intravenous pressures in the leg that occlusion of incompetent perforating veins would restore the efficiency of the particular muscle pump involved. If this occlusion is to be effected by sclerotherapy, then thrombotic blockade must be able to withstand the resultant pressures.

John Hunter is credited with the first accurate description of thrombophlebitis, in 1793. Virchow extended this to a description of the sequence of events leading to thrombosis, introducing the term "phlebothrombosis".

In the past, two types of venous thrombosis were recognised: (1) thrombophlebitis, resulting from inflammation of the vein caused by injury or by neighbouring inflammation of the vein, and (2) phlebothrombosis, a primary condition related to haemodynamic and coagulation alterations. Today, this distinction is recognised to be more theoretical than practical since in most cases the initial problem is phlebothrombosis and the thrombus itself causes inflammatory reactions in the wall of the affected vein, manifested by local and systemic signs and symptoms of an inflammatory state.

The terms are confusing, and in older literature the term "thrombophlebitis" was synonymous with superficial vein thrombosis while the term "phlebothrombosis" related to DVT. Currently, two terms are used in the British literature: DVT and superficial thrombophlebitis. Sticking to these two terms eliminates confusion.

Intravenous Thrombus

The fate of a thrombus depends on several factors, which are discussed later. In brief, a thrombus may:

- propagate and eventually cause obstruction;
- give rise to an embolus and thus be carried away in part or in whole from its site of origin;
- be removed by fibrinolytic action;
- become organised and subsequently may recanalise.

Lysis

The fibrinolytic system provides a critically important mechanism for the dissolution of fibrin clots. The major enzymes capable of digesting fibrin are leucocyte-derived proteases and plasmin. The proteolytic conversion of plasminogen, a normal plasma protein, to plasmin is accomplished either by a factor XII-dependent pathology or by well-characterised plasminogen activators. There are two distinct groups of plasminogen activators: urokinase, present in plasma and various tissues, activates plasminogen in the fluid phase, while tissue-type plasminogen activator, whose principal site of synthesis is the endothelial cell, is active when attached to fibrin. Once released, the fibrin-split products serve as potent anticoagulants.

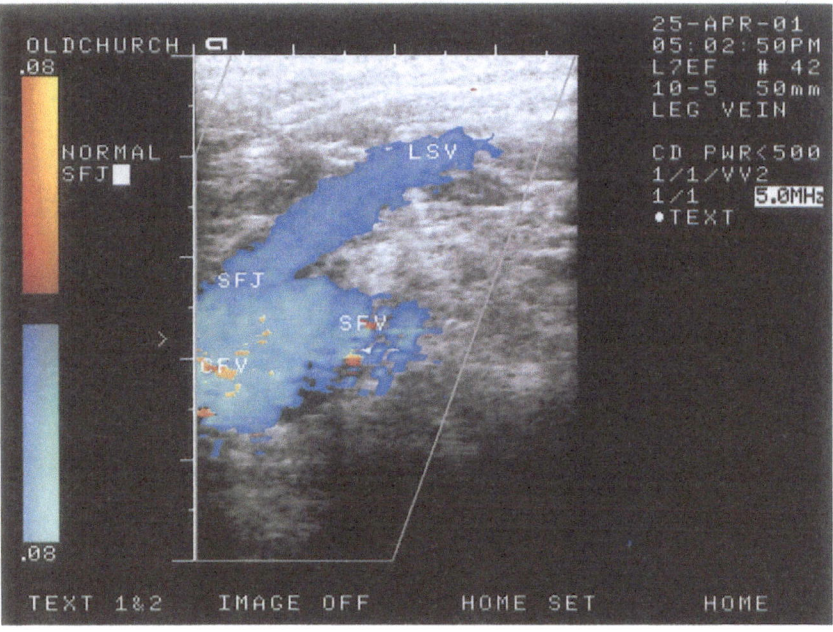

Figure 4.1 Normal saphenofemoral junction (SFJ), long saphenous vein (LSV), superficial femoral vein (SFV), and common femoral vein (CFV).

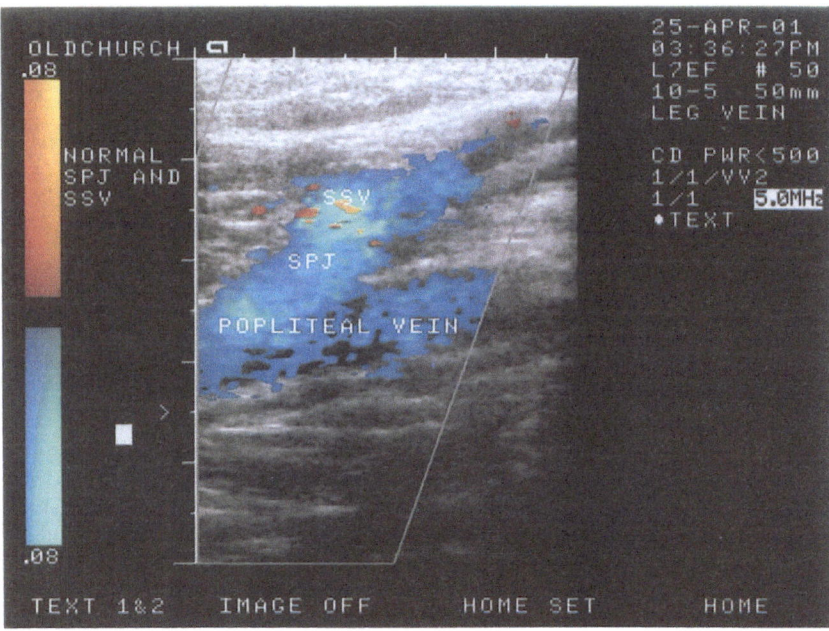

Figure 4.2 Normal saphenopopliteal junction (SPJ), short saphenous vein (SSV), and popliteal vein.

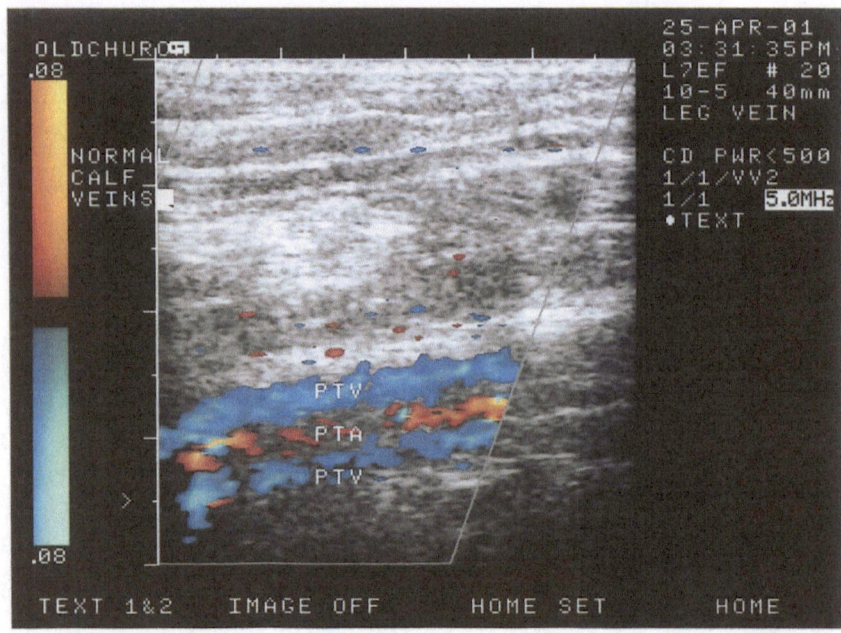

Figure 4.3 Normal posterior tibial artery (PTA) and paired posterior tibial veins (PTV).

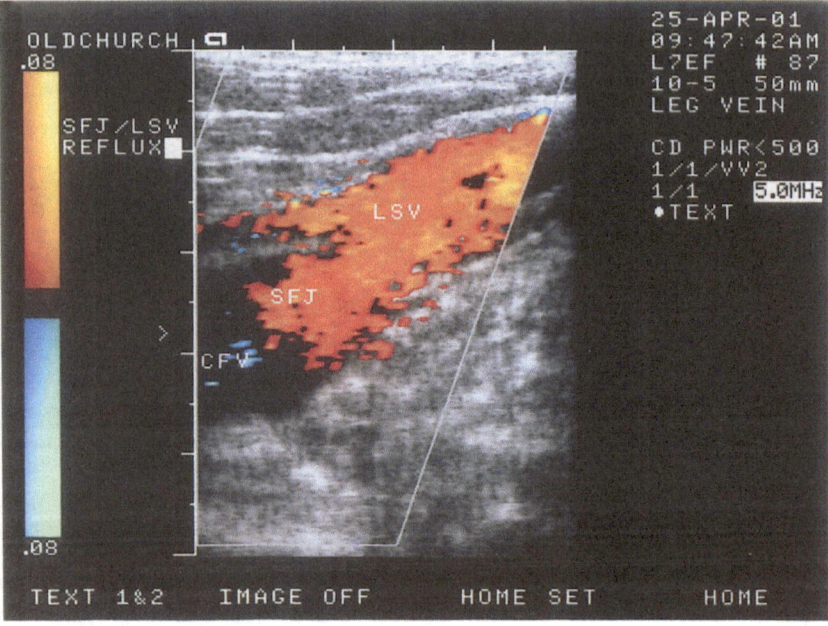

Figure 4.4 Reflux (red is set as reverse flow) in saphenofemoral junction (SFJ) and long saphenous vein (SFV). CFV, common femoral vein.

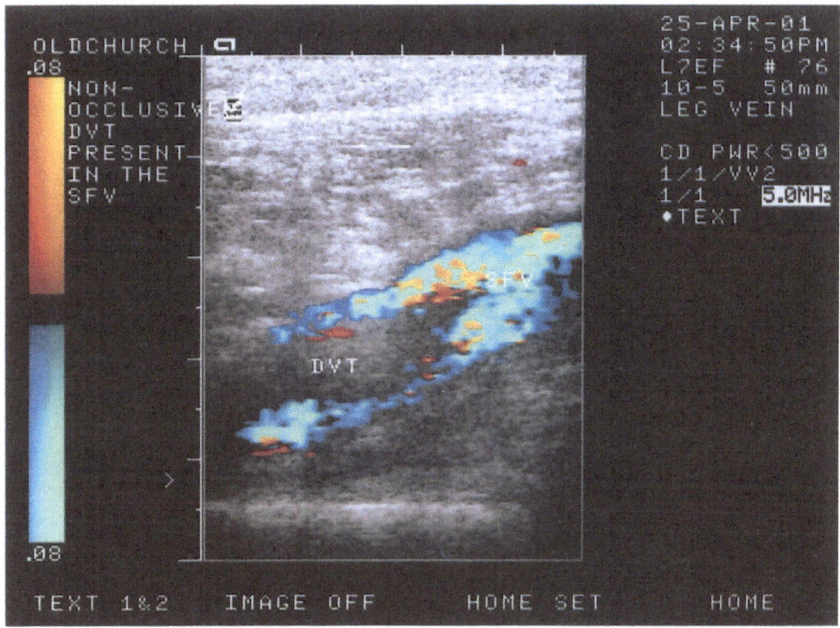

Figure 4.5 Deep venous thrombosis (DVT; appears as filling defect) in superficial femoral vein (SFV).

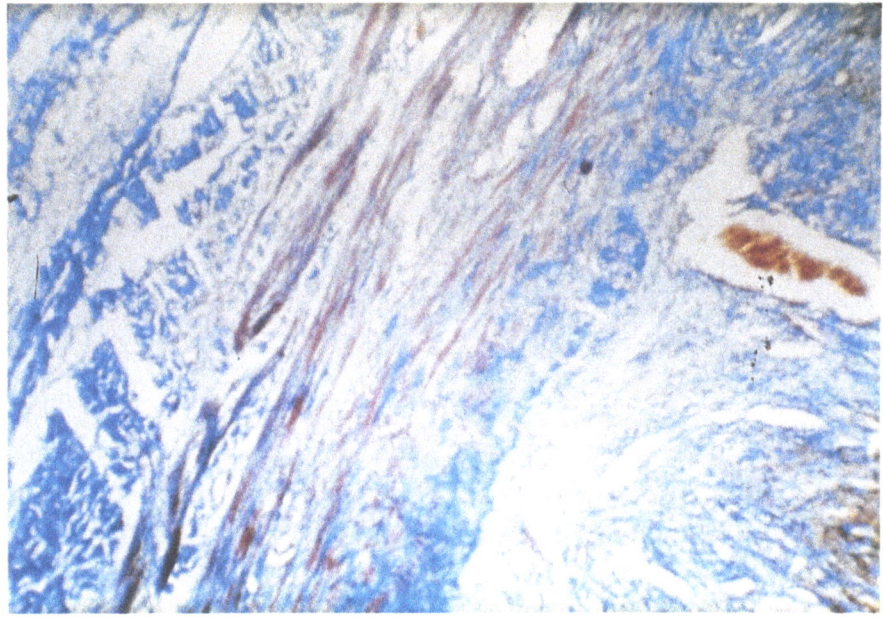

Figure 6.1 Capillaries crossing the internal elastic lamina.

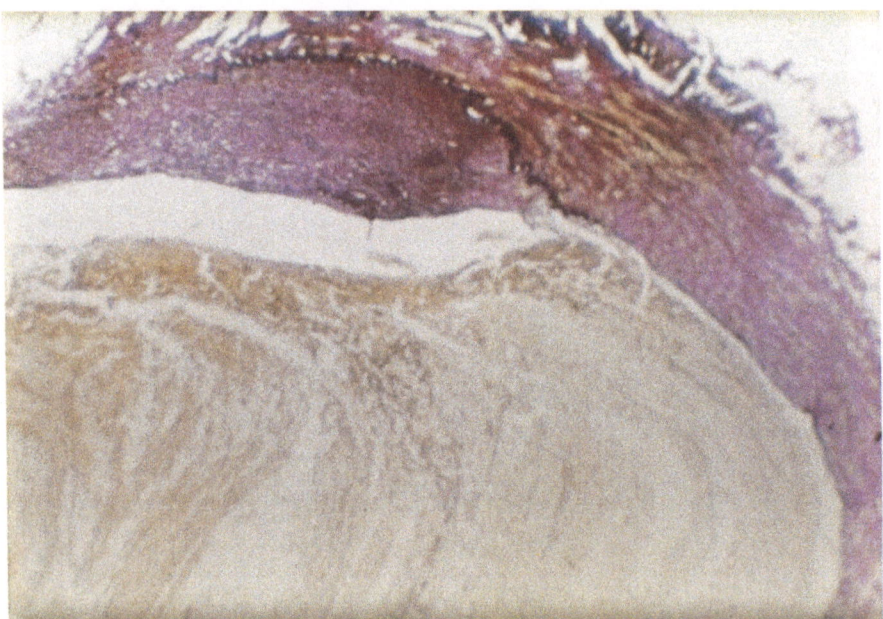

Figure 6.2 Photomicrograph of transverse section of vein affected by acute thrombophlebitis, demonstrating a relatively thin vein wall compared with the diameter of the thrombus.

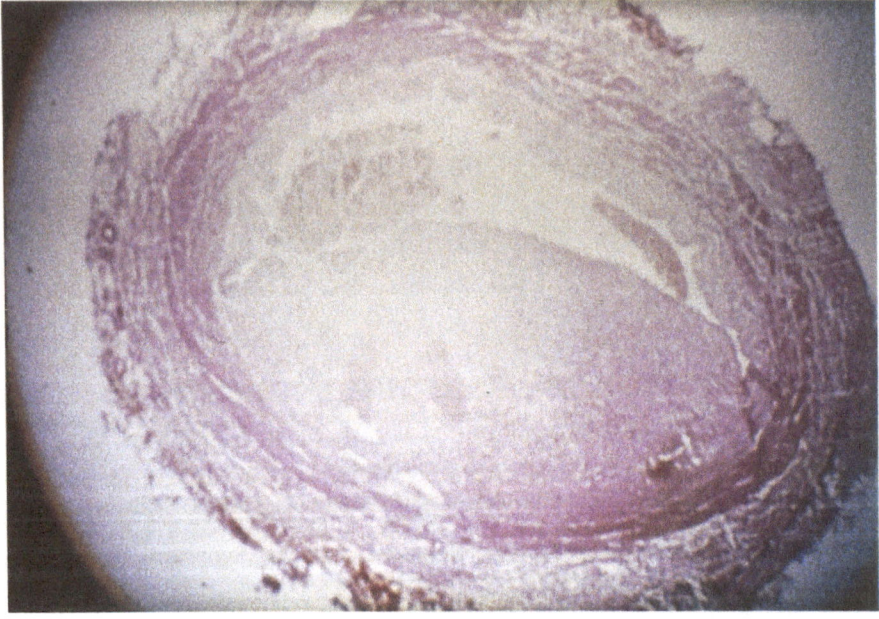

Figure 6.3 Photomicrograph showing the early development of peripheral sinuses between the thrombus and the vein wall.

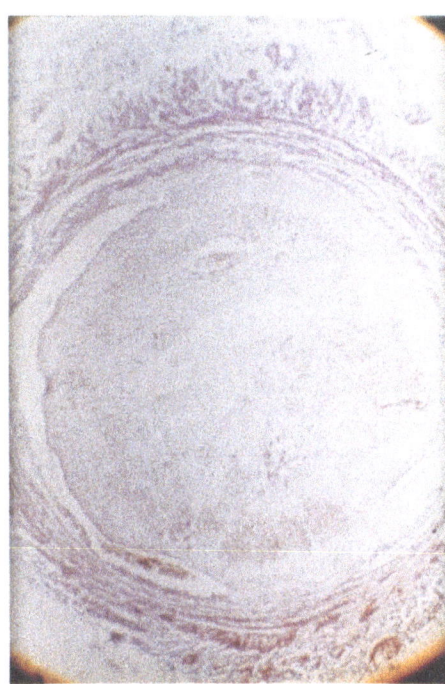

Figure 6.4 Photomicrograph showing later stage in development of peripheral sinuses. One sinus communicates with the lumen of the vein and contains blood.

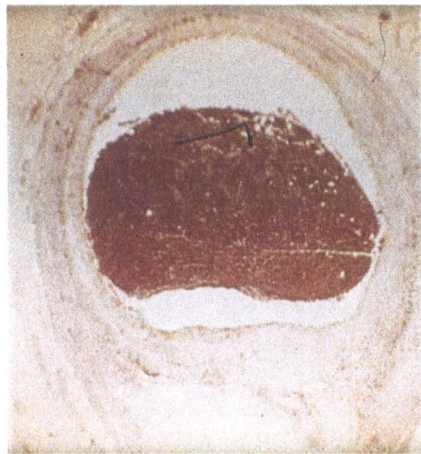

Figure 6.5 Photomicrograph showing complete recanalisation, with incorporation of the thrombus into the vein wall.

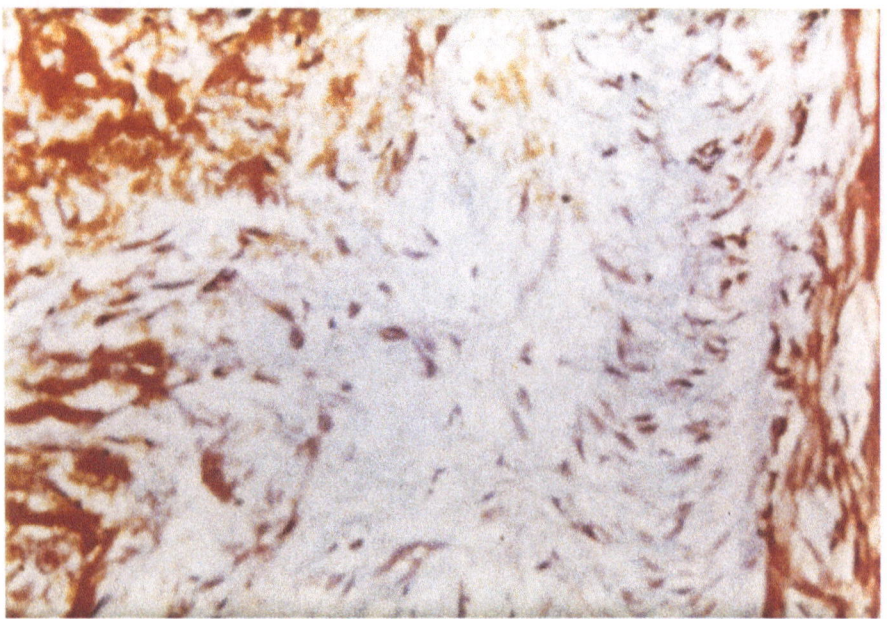

Figure 6.6 Sclerosis, showing cells from the vein wall at lower right invading the thrombus at upper left.

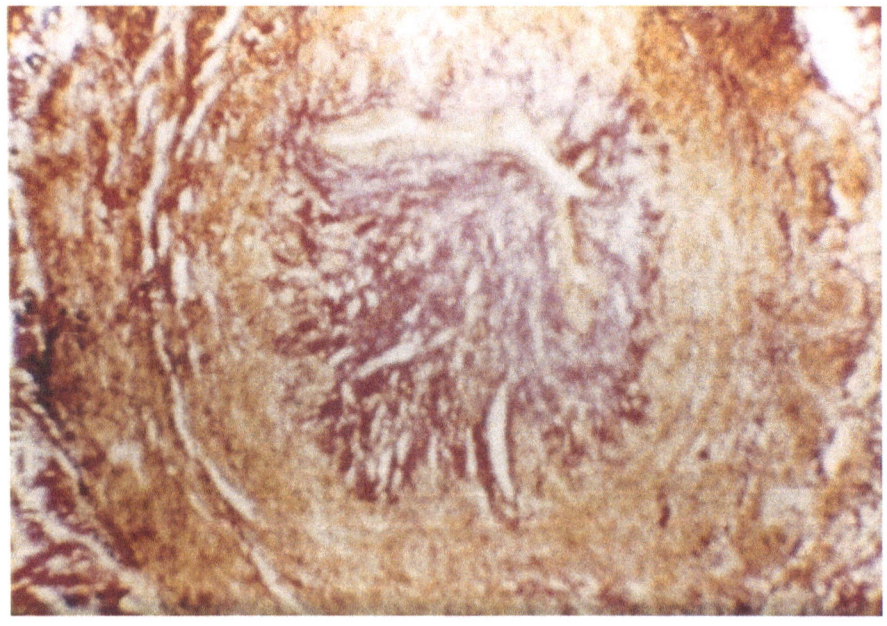

Figure 6.7 Sclerosis, showing organisation of thrombus.

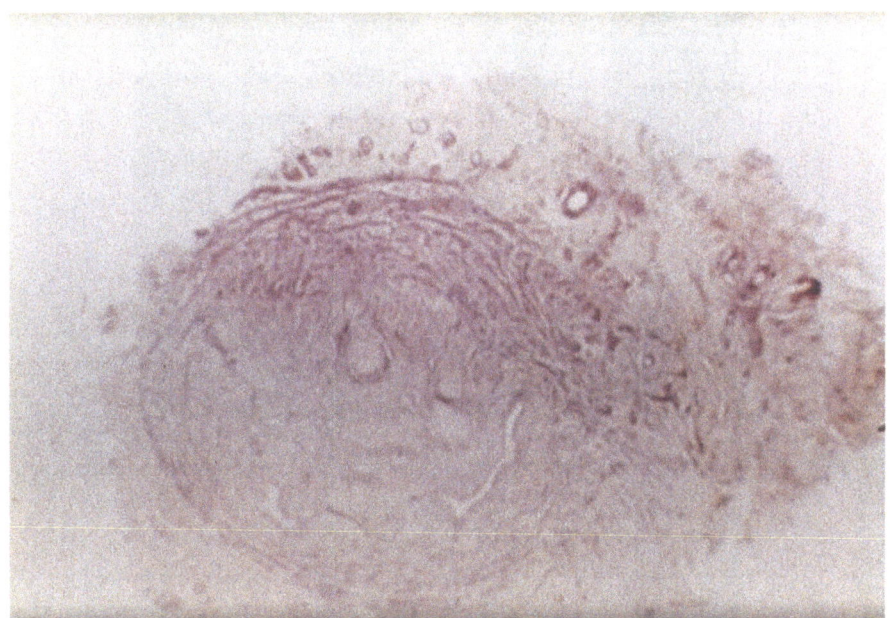

Figure 6.8 Sclerosis, showing completely organised thrombus.

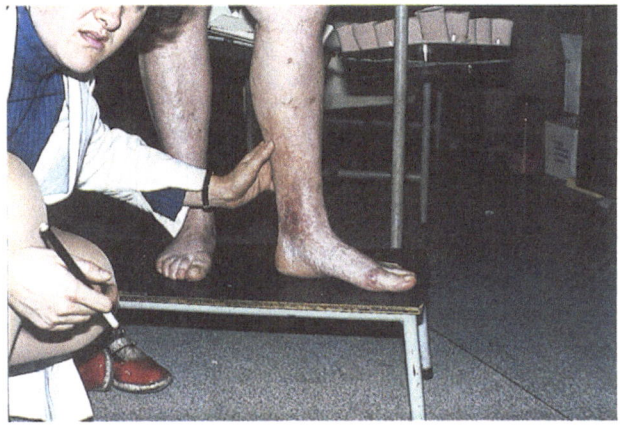

Figure 7.1 Patient standing ready to be marked.

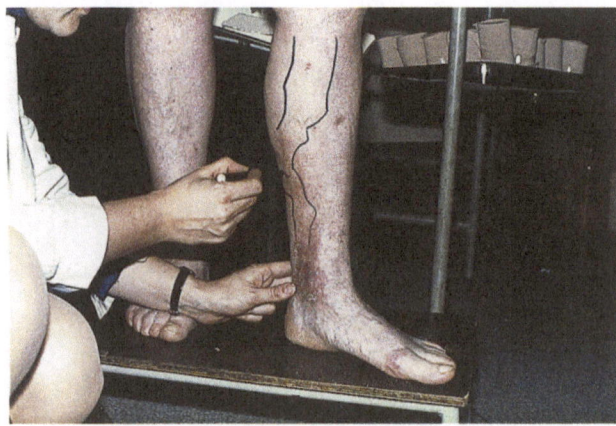

Figure 7.2 Dilated veins marked out following examination by inspection, palpation and percussion.

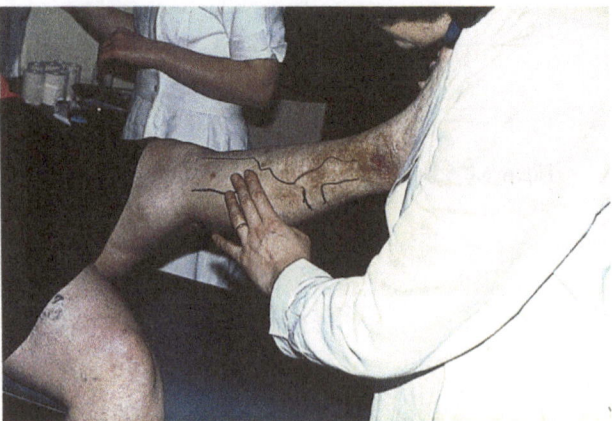

Figure 7.3 Patient lying down with the leg raised and the fascial orifices marked out, and the doctor palpating the raised leg.

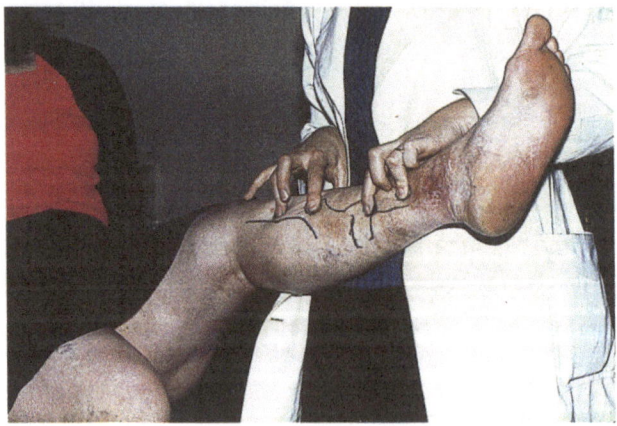

Figure 7.4 Doctor's fingers placed in fascial orifices with the patient's leg raised.

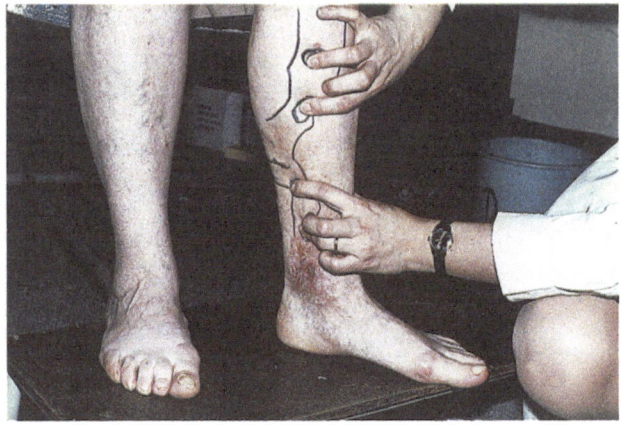

Figure 7.5 Filling of veins being controlled, with the patient standing, by finger pressure on fascial orifices.

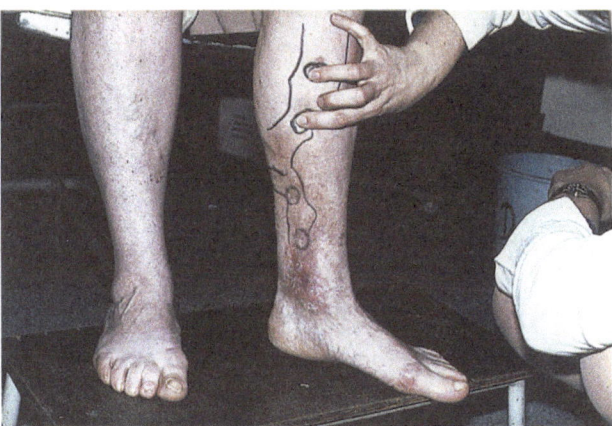

Figure 7.6 Removal of two fingers: veins do not fill.

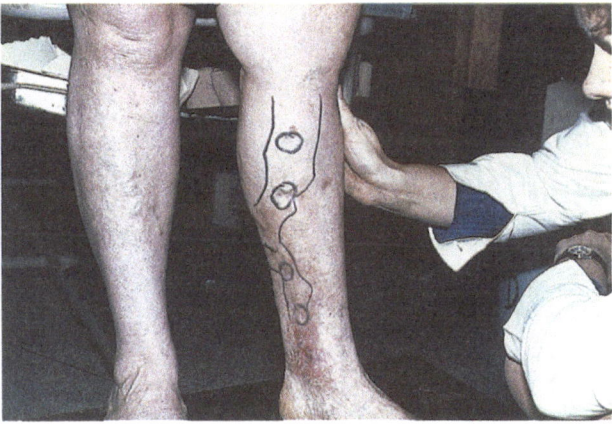

Figure 7.7 Removal of remaining fingers: veins fill.

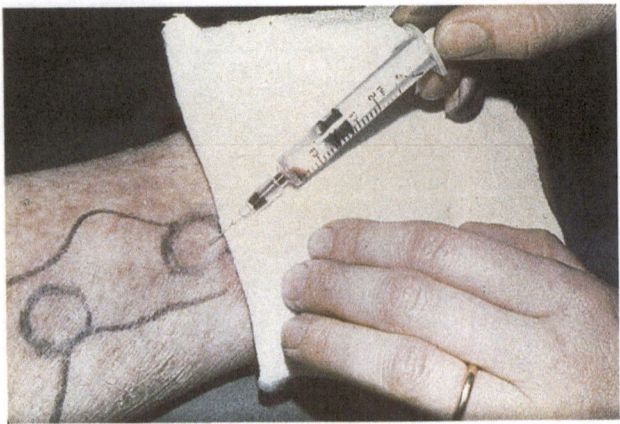

Figure 7.8 The needle is inserted into the vein while the patient sits on a couch.

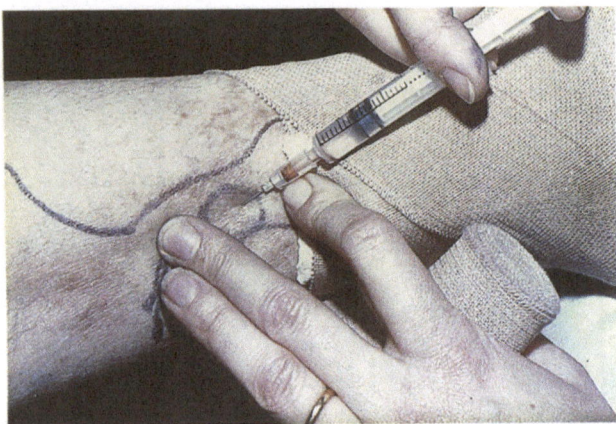

Figure 7.9 The leg is raised and the injection is given into a segment of vein isolated by firm compression by the ring and index fingers.

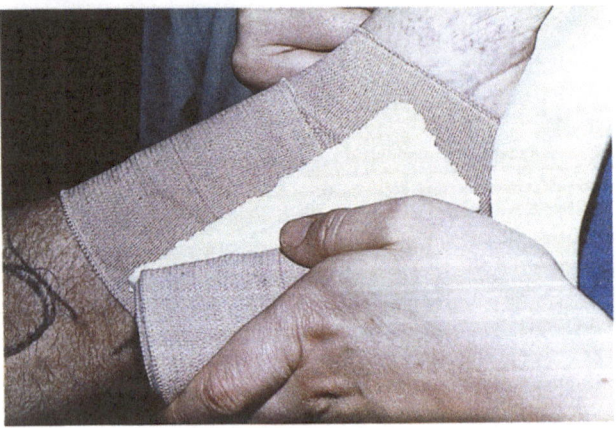

Figure 7.10 A sorbo pad is bandaged into position over the injection site.

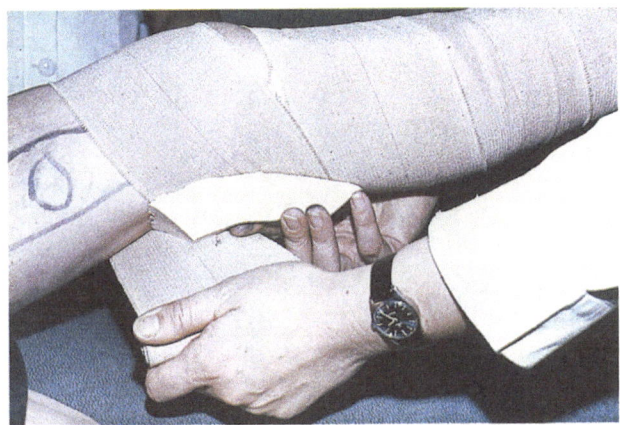

Figure 7.11 A rubber pad is placed behind the knee to prevent the bandages from rolling up and abrading the skin.

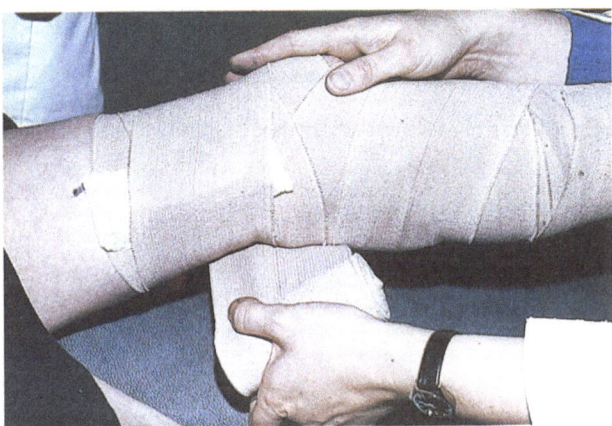

Figure 7.12 A rubber pad is left protruding above the upper edge of the bandages, preventing them from rolling down and forming a sharp ring, which would tend to traumatise the long saphenous vein and cause superficial thrombophlebitis.

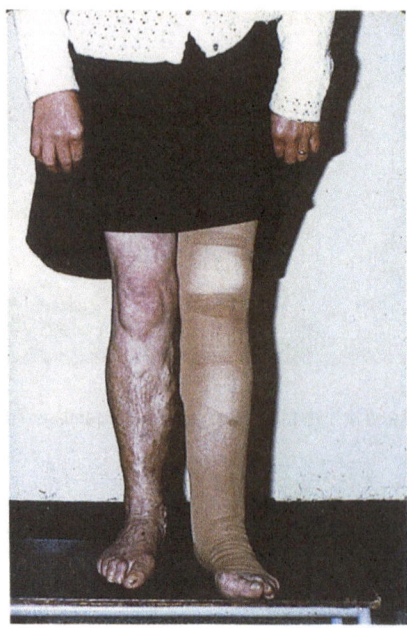

Figure 7.13 When bandaging is complete, an elastic stocking is applied and attached to a suspender belt.

It has been shown in experimental animals that the intravenous administration of plasmin or plasminogen activator will speed up the reabsorption of fresh coagulation thrombi. Plasminogen is adsorbed on to fibrin during clot formation, so subsequent lysis may be a local phenomenon occurring within the thrombus. It is also probable that the vein wall liberates highly lytic substances. Lysis may be assisted further by the ischaemia within the thrombus, causing a release of tissue activator. Enzymes released by degenerating leucocytes trapped within the thrombus may also have a lytic effect.

The fate of a thrombus that does not undergo lysis depends upon the following factors:

- The ratio of the diameter of the thrombus to the thickness of the surrounding vein wall. This ratio may vary at different regions of the same specimen.
- The degree of cellular activity in the vein wall, and the rapidity with which it develops.
- The degree of cellular and capillary invasion of the thrombus.
- The intravenous pressure and the degree of fluctuation of pressure in the vein above and below the area of phlebitis.

These factors are important because they determine the rate and completeness of organisation and the degree to which recanalisation takes place.

Organisation

This is a process by which the thrombus is invaded by cellular elements – leucocytes, fibroblasts and capillaries – from the vein wall. The thrombus becomes attached firmly to the vein wall where this occurs. Microscopic examination of sections of veins involved in thrombophlebitis shows that the vasa vasorum in the intima and media are considerably dilated and new capillaries derived from these vessels cross the vein wall, traverse the internal elastic lamina (Figure 6.1), and invade the thrombus.

This cellular activity appears to be associated with trauma to the intima of the vein. The greater the area of intimal damage, the greater will be the area over which

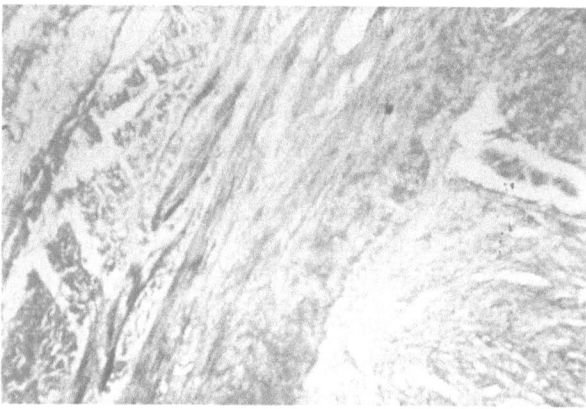

Figure 6.1 Capillaries crossing the internal elastic lamina. Also Plate III.

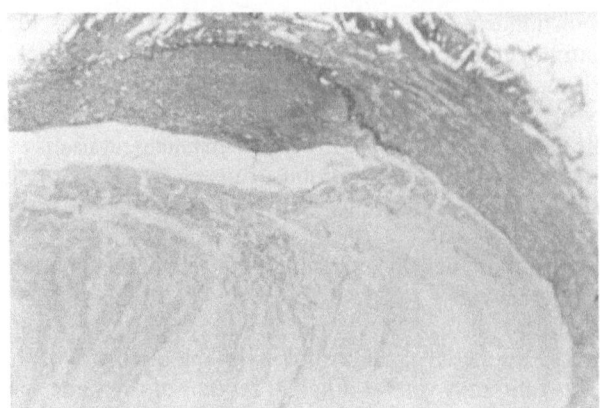

Figure 6.2 Photomicrograph of transverse section of vein affected by acute thrombophlebitis, demonstrating a relatively thin vein wall compared with the diameter of the thrombus. Also Plate IV.

cellular activity develops. Cellular activity is more pronounced in a contracted thick wall than in one that is stretched and thin. This may be because the nutrition of a dilated vein is impaired.

Recanalisation

The first essential step in recanalisation is the development of slit-like sinuses between the thrombus and the vein wall. These sinuses are infrequent and remain small in areas where invasion of the thrombus from the vein wall is taking place. If the thrombus is subjected to pressures from above, below and via the perforating veins, then the sinuses enlarge and coalesce and recanalisation occurs.

Fibrosis

Fibrosis ultimately occurs in those areas of the thrombus that have undergone organisation. Vascularisation promotes the development of collagen. As the collagen matures, the capillary network regresses. The vein wall itself does not become fibrosed completely, but there is an increase in collagen separating the muscle fibres in continuity with the collagen in the thrombus. Deposits of haemosiderin may be found in parts of the vein wall, in the fibrosed thrombus, and in the perivenous tissue.

In order to illustrate the sequelae of thrombophlebitis more clearly, we will describe two extreme examples: (1) phlebitis in which a large-diameter thrombus develops with a thin, distended vein wall encircling it, and (2) phlebitis in which a relatively small-diameter thrombus develops within a contracted vein with a thick encircling vein wall, as a result of compression of the vein.

The former is the condition usually described as superficial thrombophlebitis. The lumen of the vein is fully occupied by clotted blood. The wall of the vein is stretched and painful. The wall/thrombus ratio is such that the diameter of the thrombus may be more than 20 times the thickness of the vein wall (Figure 6.2).

During the first 48 hours, cellular activity occurs over most of the intima. One or two areas soon predominate, and invading cells stream into the thrombus from these

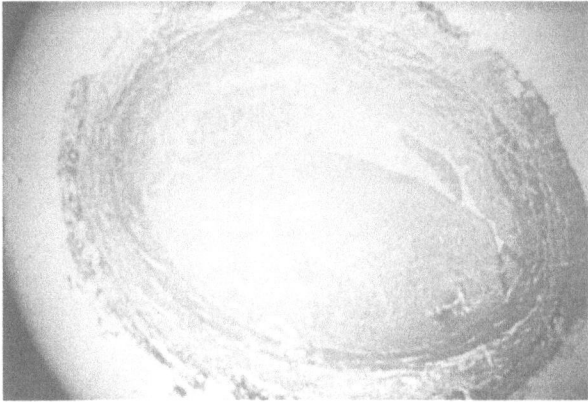

Figure 6.3 Photomicrograph showing the early development of peripheral sinuses between the thrombus and the vein wall. Also Plate IV.

points. The invasion is not very aggressive and takes place from a relatively small area of the intima. Because of the large diameter of the thrombus, the central part undergoes degeneration before the invading cellular elements can reach it. Recanalisation commences, with the appearance of peripheral sinuses between the thrombus and the vein wall (Figure 6.3). The thrombus is subjected to high pressures and the slit-like sinuses gradually dilate and coalesce (Figure 6.4). The thrombus itself undergoes fibrosis and may ultimately be surrounded by several channels, or it may be displaced to one side and included in the vein wall (Figure 6.5). The end result of this type of thrombosis is therefore recanalisation. In addition, if the thrombosis takes place in an area in which there are normal valves, then these will be destroyed.

Phlebitis in which a relatively small-diameter thrombus develops within a contracted vein with a thick encircling vein wall occurs when the technique of compression sclerotherapy is used successfully. The empty-vein technique ensures the presence of only a minimal amount of blood in the vein. Isolation of the segment of vein prevents extension of the thrombosis beyond the selected area and, as the sclerosant is undiluted by blood, most of the intima within this area is severely damaged. The vein wall is thick and contracted and consequently profuse cellular activity takes place over a relatively wide area of intima (Figure 6.6). Compression of the vein and ambulation of the patient protect the thrombus from pulsatile pressures. The small-diameter thrombus is therefore invaded rapidly and widely, and there is little opportunity for recanalisation to occur (Figure 6.7). The thrombus subsequently undergoes fibrosis and remains firmly attached around most of its periphery to the surrounding vein wall (Figure 6.8). This process is described in detail below.

Histological Changes at Varying Times after Injection and Application of Compression

It is clear that the technique of emptying the vein and applying finger compression above and below the segment selected for injection does not succeed in emptying the

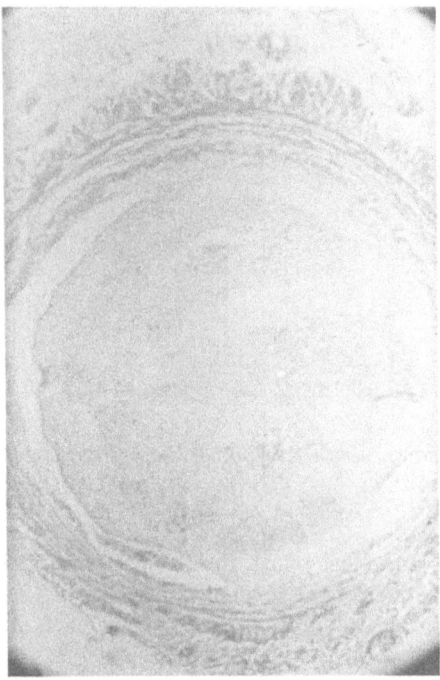

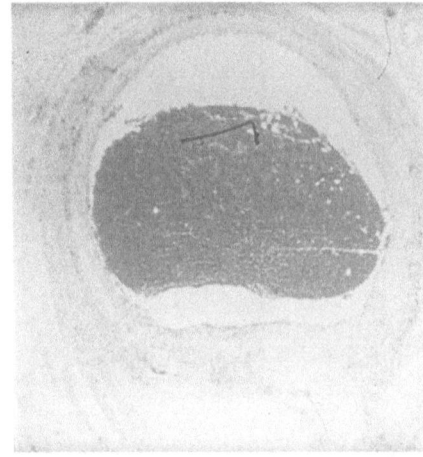

Figure 6.5 Photomicrograph showing complete recanalisation, with incorporation of the thrombus into the vein wall. Also Plate V.

Figure 6.4 Photomicrograph showing later stage in development of peripheral sinuses. One sinus communicates with the lumen of the vein and contains blood. Also Plate V.

vein entirely. Thirty seconds after injection, a varying amount of blood is left in the lumen. The following changes are observed: Over most of the circumference of the vessel, the endothelial lining cells have disappeared completely, or been cast into the lumen, or remain in position. In each case, they are altered as follows: the cells have rounded up and are swollen, the nuclei are enlarged, and the chromatin is coarsely granular or irregularly clumped, suggesting the early stages of karyorrhexis. Where a number of cells remain attached side by side to form a row, a jagged, uneven, saw-tooth appearance is seen instead of the usual smooth lining common to endothelial surfaces. This is caused by the apparent disintegration of the cement lines between cells, which appear partly or completely detached one from the other, while remaining individually attached, at least for the present, at the base. All are swollen, and some project further than others into the lumen, while some are unusually tall and stand up in a peg-like fashion with the nucleus at the luminal border. The small quantity of blood remaining in the lumen (when compression is good) shows agglutinated masses of red blood cells alternating with paler pink areas of a fine fibrin network. Fibrin is clinging to the denuded endothelial surfaces and also to areas of surviving but altered endothelium. Some masses of agglutinated red cells lying in close proximity to these surfaces show the presence of large numbers of readily distinguishable platelets. It is not unreasonable to postulate a sequence of events in which, following chemical damage to the endothelium, platelets are attracted to these surfaces and adhere both to the surface and to each other, thus initiating the clotting process that involves any blood lying in the lumen of the vein segment.

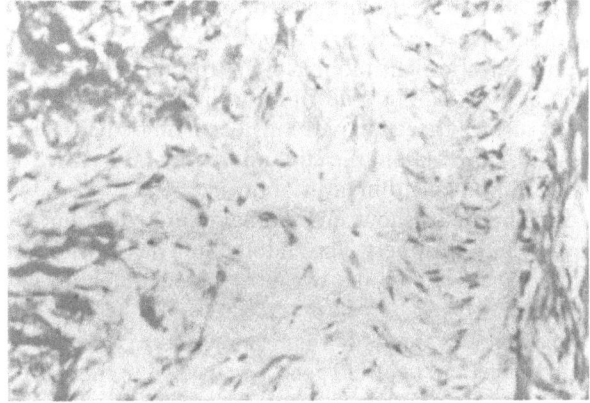

Figure 6.6 Sclerosis, showing cells from the vein wall at lower right invading the thrombus at upper left. Also Plate VI.

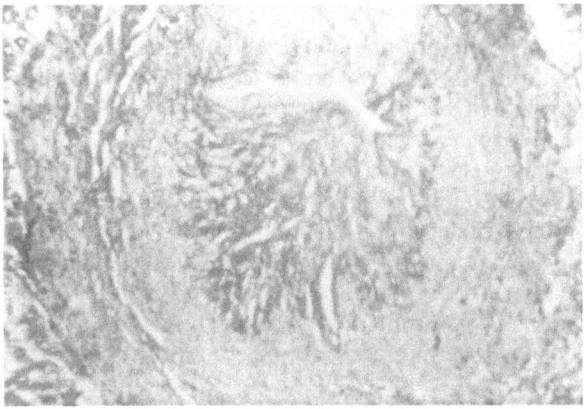

Figure 6.7 Sclerosis, showing organisation of thrombus. Also Plate VI.

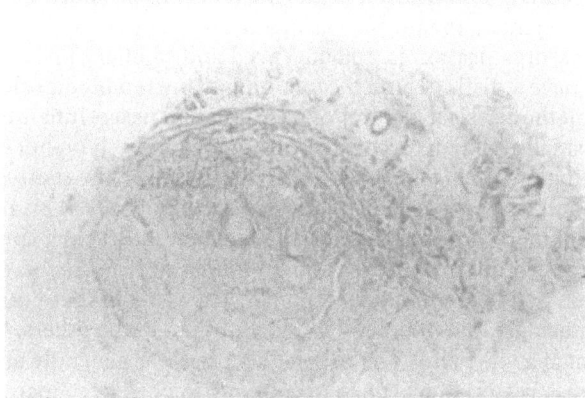

Figure 6.8 Sclerosis, showing completely organised thrombus. Also Plate VII.

One minute after injection, the number of endothelial cells still in position is reduced further; otherwise, there is no change.

Twelve hours after injection, the blood clot has the appearance of being formed in a standing column of blood and is a fibrin/red-cell complex. There is no evidence of layering of the clot, such as is seen in naturally occurring DVT. The endothelium has disappeared from most areas about the circumference of the vessel, and the resulting denuded areas are covered by a thin layer of fibrin.

At 24 hours, the blood clot shows numerous fissures distributed irregularly but found mainly towards the periphery. The endothelium has mostly disappeared about the entire circumference. The amount of surviving endothelium seen varies somewhat from vein to vein.

At 36 hours, the commencement of organisation of the clot is seen. At a number of points (usually not more than two, and generally located in the same quadrant of the circumference), distinct finger-like processes consisting of proliferating fibroblasts can be seen advancing into the clot. The time at which organisation begins seems to vary substantially. In some biopsies examined, no attempt at organisation was observed, even after a lapse of five days. No cause, clinical or morphological, could be ascertained for this.

At six days, organisation continues but is still in the early stages. Some fibroblasts, however, have by now crossed the clot and reached the opposite side. Organisation is still very limited in extent, being present at only one or two points of the circumference and not extending very far into the clot.

At 12 days, the process now appears to have accelerated. Only a small quantity of blood, apparently little altered, occupies the centre of the lumen of the vein. Outside this, there is a thick layer of fibrin extending about the entire circumference, and organising fibroblasts are moving in wide wedges from a number of points. Those coming from the same quadrant may join laterally with one another.

At 14 days, fibroblasts in proliferating wedges, spreading from opposite or near-opposite points of the circumference, are meeting in the centre of the vessel. Any blood still remaining in the lumen is usually pushed to one side. Note that at this point, for the first time, active new capillary formation is proceeding. Thus, we can assume up to two weeks elapse before the vascularisation stage of organisation begins in these cases. In all the cases observed up to this point, compression of the vein had been good. If compression is playing a part in promoting eventual fibrous obliteration of a segment, then it is clear that it cannot be relaxed at this stage.

At three weeks, organisation is well advanced and capillary formation is marked. The capillaries have a distinct lumen containing many red blood cells. The organising clot shows all the classical features of a granulation tissue. Inflammatory cells are scanty, with a small number of polymorphs, rather more lymphocytes, and a few plasma cells being present. Even at this late stage, however, the centre of the original thrombus may still show apparently unaffected red blood cells. This may in fact represent a trickle of blood passing through the segment rather than surviving cells.

Biopsy was carried out at four weeks on a number of cases where it was known that compression had been maintained poorly. The veins in these cases showed the presence of a much greater volume of blood clot than in the others. Early organisation was evident at a few points on the periphery but was generally at an early stage. By way of contrast, vessels in which good compression had been maintained without interruption showed a picture of very good organisation, with bands of proliferating fibroblasts crossing the lumen in its entire width and advanced capillary formation.

By seven weeks, it is clear that the desired end result is being achieved. The vascular granulation tissue described above is replaced by young cellular fibrous tissue, which fills most of the lumen of the vessel. It should be noted that in these vessels, the lumen is far smaller when good compression has been maintained without interruption than when compression has been poor. The amount of space requiring to be filled by fibrous tissue is thus considerably less, and it is not surprising that the majority of these veins show almost total obliteration by young fibrous tissue. At seven weeks, most vessels show one or more re-established vascular channels lined by regenerated endothelium, through which blood is obviously flowing. These channels are small, however, and the clinical results obtained in these cases would suggest that they are not significant.

At ten weeks, the fibrous tissue is still a young cellular tissue containing numerous plump fibroblasts: capillaries are still evident but becoming less prominent. Small peripheral sinuses lined by endothelium are present at one or more points about the circumference. It is evident that these have formed at areas where the original blood clot has retracted from the wall of the vein between the areas of fibroblastic proliferation.

At 16 weeks, little change is seen from the previous picture. Most of the vein is occupied by vascular fibrous tissue. Many veins do not show the peripheral sinuses described above but are filled with fibrous tissue about their entire circumference; however, these generally show a number of central fissures or sinuses lined by endothelium and presumably in continuity with the endothelial surfaces proximal and distal to the almost totally occluded segment.

At six to seven months, the appearance is of a vessel containing mostly fibrous tissue with a number of fissure-like endothelium-lined channels present either in the centre of the vessel or towards the periphery, where presumably they are the end result of initial clot retraction and subsequent endothelialisation. It is noteworthy that the cases where the history of compression is good tend to be those where the vascular channels remaining are located more centrally in the vessel. In other words, successful compression leads to organisation all around the circumference of the vessel. It is easy to accept that this will give a better clinical result than where organisation is limited to portions of the circumference. The fibrous tissue at this stage is still quite cellular, but some collagen fibre formation is evident.

At one year, the fibrous tissue shows evidence of maturity, cellularity is diminished, and the fibroblasts present are elongated cells in contrast to the plump cells seen previously: collagen formation is proceeding.

Five years after injection compression therapy, in most cases the vein shows firm fibrosis throughout its entire circumference except for a few small irregular fissure-like channels lined by endothelium. Some vessels show hyaline change of the collagenous tissue, but in general the picture is that of well-organised fibrous tissue with gradually increasing collagen formation. The organised clot has by now become incorporated into the vein wall, forming an integral part of it.

Summary and Conclusion

Histological studies were carried out on varicose veins treated by compression sclerotherapy. The material consisted of biopsies performed on veins at intervals from 30 seconds to five years after injection. The chief purpose of the study was to observe the histological changes in varicose veins and to determine the changes occurring in the vein subsequent to therapy and to correlate such changes with the clinical results obtained. These findings can be summarised as follows:

Injection sclerotherapy produces a fibrous occlusion of the selected vein segment, which correlates well with the subsequent clinical course of the patient. The application of pressure is an essential part of the treatment and examination of the histological sequence of events in the thrombus indicates clearly that this must be maintained for at least six weeks, but preferably eight weeks, to allow that organisation to proceed to fibrous occlusion of the lumen.

No marked increase in subendothelial connective tissue occurred in the injected veins, as might have been expected when intraluminal pressure diminished. The application of external pressure may be a factor in preventing this. Varicose veins show such variation of change in the vessel wall itself, such as increased fibrosis of the media, and muscle hypertrophy and atrophy, that it is not easy to determine from a study of biopsies of injected veins whether changes in the wall are associated with therapy or whether they preceded it. Further study of the vein wall and perivenous tissues is required.

In some biopsies of injected veins, no attempt at clot organisation was evident even five days after injection. The cause of this delay did not emerge during the course of the study. In general, organisation of the clot produced is quite slow: it is clear that up to two weeks elapse before the vascularisation stage of organisation is produced. It is not surprising that most previous attempts at injection of varicose veins ended in failure, as any clots formed were rapidly recanalised or lysed completely. Compression maintained without interruption is essential to promote good organisation of the clot. Furthermore, successful compression leads to organisation all around the circumference of the vessel, which in turn produces the best and most enduring clinical results.

Properties and Action of Sodium Tetradecyl Sulphate

The sclerosant used in the form of treatment described in this book is sodium tetradecyl sulphate (sodium 1-isobutyl-4-ethyloctyl sulphate). It is the salt of an alkali metal and a long-chain fatty acid, and so it has the properties of a soap. In its solid state, it is a white, waxy substance that is soluble in water, alcohol and ether. A 3% solution in 2% benzyl alcohol is prepared for clinical use.

Effects of Sodium Tetradecyl Sulphate on Blood in Vitro

Haemolysis

Varying concentrations of sodium tetradecyl sulphate in normal saline were added to heparinised blood. Fragility curves were plotted, with the following results:

- Red blood cells were lysed at sodium tetradecyl sulphate concentrations of 0.125% or greater.
- White blood cells were lysed at sodium tetradecyl sulphate concentrations of 0.1% or greater.
- Disruption of the membranes occurred at a concentration of 0.05%.

Denaturation of Serum Proteins

Addition of sodium tetradecyl sulphate to serum caused turbidity. Subsequent electrophoresis of this serum showed abnormal migration of the protein fractions. The reaction, which is very rapid, appears to be a combination of sodium tetradecyl sulphate and plasma protein. As a result, there is complete inhibition of the detergent properties of the sclerosant.

Effects of Sodium Tetradecyl Sulphate on Blood in Vivo

In a study of ten patients, blood and urine samples were taken just before and 45 minutes after intravenous injections of sodium tetradecyl sulphate. Each patient received 1.5–3 ml sodium tetradecyl sulphate as part of the treatment for varicose veins. The bleeding time was measured, and the following investigations were performed on the blood samples:

- clotting time;
- prothrombin time;
- thromboplastin generation test;
- platelet count;
- serum direct van den Berg reaction;
- serum bilirubin estimation;
- serum glutamic oxalacetic transaminase estimation;
- serum glutamic pyruvic transaminase estimation;
- lactic dehydrogenase estimation.

Spectroscopic examination for methaemoglobin and methalbumin was also performed. The samples of urine were investigated for abnormal deposits, albumin and urobilinogen.

Apart from a slight increase in platelets in seven patients, the injection of sodium tetradecyl sulphate produced no changes in the results of any of these tests.

Effects of Sodium Tetradecyl Sulphate on Blood Clotting in Vitro

A solution of 0.05% sodium tetradecyl sulphate in normal saline was used to reconstitute dried fibrinogen, thromboplastin or thrombin. Thromboplastin generation tests were then performed. Sodium tetradecyl sulphate prevented the formation of a fibrous clot in each case, regardless of which constituent it had been added to.

Effects of Intravenous Injection of Benzyl Alcohol

Since the solution of sodium tetradecyl sulphate used clinically contains 2% benzyl alcohol, it was important to discover the active agent in producing local endosclerosis. A small series of intravenous injections of 2% benzyl alcohol solution followed by compression and ambulation, as in the technique described in this book, failed to produce any clinical evidence of a sclerotic action at the site of injection.

Conclusions from in Vitro Experiments

Sodium tetradecyl sulphate combines rapidly with and denatures protein, causes haemolysis in vitro, and inhibits blood coagulation.

Suggested Mode of Action of Sodium Tetradecyl Sulphate

These results suggest that the thrombus appearing at the injection site is not due to the action of sodium tetradecyl sulphate on blood. Sodium tetradecyl sulphate probably combines with the protein of the endothelial lining, damaging the intimal cells. Normal blood subsequently clots on the damaged intima. This explanation is supported by the clinical belief that an injection is more likely to be successful if the vein is empty of blood at the time of injection, since any blood present would tend to inactivate the sodium tetradecyl sulphate. It would also explain why involvement of the deep veins is so rare, since any sclerosant spilling into the deep system would be inactivated by the contained blood.

7 Compression Sclerotherapy: Theory, Method and Practice

G. Fegan

In compression sclerotherapy, reverse flow in the perforating veins between the deep and superficial veins is located. The veins at these sites are then obliterated permanently by the injection of a sclerosant, which initiates controlled thrombosis, and by the application of continuous pressure. The technique relies on the restoration of the pumping capacity of the multiple muscle pumps of the foot, calf and thigh, rather than on the eradication of superficial varices or the opening up of proximal obstruction. Advantage is also taken of the fact that not all incompetent valves are injured permanently. Valves may be incompetent because the vein containing them is dilated (secondary incompetence); they can regain normal function when the vein reduces in size after the efficiency of the pumps is restored and normal ambulatory venous pressure achieved. It is unnecessary to be so radical as to strip out superficial veins, or to thrombose them along their entire length by indiscriminate multiple injections. The proximal half of the LSV is one of the best "spare parts" that human beings carry, and it should not be stripped out without good reason.

Attention is directed first to the most distal leaks from the deep system. The proximal dilated veins are then watched for improvements; a surprising degree of resolution often takes place in a grossly dilated tortuous vein above the knee following the restoration of the efficiency of the pumps of the foot and calf. Even large saphena varices often disappear within a few weeks of treatment of a perforating vein in the calf.

It should be appreciated that there is usually a large physiological reserve in the lower limb, and that considerable damage must be done before the signs and symptoms of venous insufficiency appear. Conversely, it is unnecessary to restore the pumps completely to normal in order to relieve congestion and effect clinical cures. In fact, if complete and perfect restoration of the pumps were essential for successful treatment, then few patients would ever be cured by any form of treatment.

Selection of Patients

Selection of patients is carried out for two reasons: to find those with no indication for compression sclerotherapy, and to reject those with some contraindication to it. Patients are occasionally referred for treatment of signs and symptoms that are not actually due to CVI of the lower limb. The commonest conditions found in these patients are orthopaedic causes of pain in the lower limb, arterial disease, oedema of systemic nature, erythrocyanosis frigida, and non-varicose leg ulcers. Frequently, one of these conditions coexists with CVI, and in such cases it must be explained to the patient that treatment of the veins will not give complete relief from the symptoms.

Contraindications to Compression Sclerotherapy

The contraindications to compression sclerotherapy are:

- *Fat legs:* It is essential that the bandages applied immediately after the injection stay in place for up to six weeks. If the patient's legs are fat, then the bandages cannot be applied satisfactorily. It is also very difficult to find the perforating veins in fat legs. Such patients are advised to lose weight before treatment is started. If a varicose ulcer is present, however, compression over the ulcer is applied immediately and maintained as well as possible.
- *Inability to walk:* Walking for an hour every day is very important in the treatment. If the patient is unable to do this, e.g. due to paralysis, arthritis, cardiopulmonary disease, or confinement to bed, then treatment should not be undertaken.
- *Acute cellulitis:* Injections should not be given until the acute inflammation has resolved. However, a localised area of cellulitis surrounding an ulcer is not a contraindication.
- *Veins in a site impossible to compress:* Veins above the level of mid-thigh cannot usually be compressed satisfactorily, with the exception of vulval varices. Therefore, they should not be injected.
- *Cosmetic reasons:* Caution should be exercised in the treatment of asymptomatic veins for cosmetic reasons only. Injections can cause staining of the overlying skin, which may not disappear for a year or two. Occasionally, injections cause ulcers, which leave a small scar on healing. Both will be deeply resented by the patient who seeks treatment for cosmetic reasons only. It is common for minor degrees of symptomless varices to remain unprogressive for many years in cases where pregnancy or some other aggravating cause does not intervene.
- *Hot weather:* If the weather is very hot, then the bandages and elastic stocking are liable to become very uncomfortable. It is advisable to warn patients seeking treatment during the summer of this, and in hot climates it would probably be better to undertake injection sclerotherapy only in cooler weather.
- *Allergic reactions:* A severe allergic reaction to sodium tetradecyl is an obvious contraindication to further treatment.

Except for patients with fat legs, who are encountered frequently, these contraindications arise very infrequently. Almost every patient with varicose veins can be treated by injection sclerotherapy, either immediately at the first visit or following weight reduction. Perhaps it should be emphasised that ulceration, eczema, thrombophlebitis, and a history of previous DVT are not contraindications to treatment by this method. Ulceration and eczema, however, would make surgery undesirable. The method can also be applied safely to patients suffering from systemic conditions that would make non-essential operations undesirable.

Examination

The patient is examined while standing still. The whole limb, up to and including the saphenous opening, should be exposed. It may be a minute or two before full dilation of the superficial venous system is seen (Figure 7.1). The veins are inspected, and all visible veins are marked with a skin marker.

With the patient standing, the limb is then palpated. This will often reveal further veins, and these too are marked. A large dilated vein is now percussed while the limb is palpated. The percussion thrill can often be felt for considerable distances along veins that are otherwise undetectable. These veins are also marked (Figure 7.2).

The patient now sits down on a couch, then lies back with the legs hanging over the end of the couch. The limb being examined is raised and, with the muscles relaxed, the heel is rested on the doctor's shoulder or chest. The limb is then palpated thoroughly with both hands. The limb in this position feels strikingly different from the limb of the standing patient. The veins are empty, the muscles are relaxed, and the whole limb is much softer. The leg should be examined by applying the hands to the leg, with the fingers slightly flexed and moving the hands fairly rapidly up and down the leg. Palpation of the raised leg is carried out in order to detect orifices in the deep fascia. It is through such orifices that incompetent perforating veins pass. These orifices may be felt as definite openings with a sharp edge all round, or as areas of abnormal softness. A space in the superficial fascia produced by a varix of the superficial vein may give a very similar feeling, and is very difficult to distinguish by palpation from an opening in the deep fascia unless one has had considerable experience. However, they can be distinguished by a further test.

All the suspected fascial orifices are marked with a skin marker (Figure 7.3). The most likely sites of retrograde filling can be chosen by considering the relation of the suspected fascial orifices to the marked complex of superficial veins and the known sites of perforating veins.

As many as possible of the likely sites of retrograde filling are compressed with the tips of the doctor's fingers (Figure 7.4), and the patient then stands up. With the compression maintained, the limb is watched for filling of the superficial veins (Figure 7.5). If this occurs, the test is repeated with pressure placed on different sites. Once filling of the superficial veins is controlled by the pressure of the fingertips on a few sites, the fingers are removed one by one (Figure 7.6). When the finger is withdrawn from an orifice that is transmitting a perforating vein, the valve of which is incompetent, the superficial veins fill slowly (Figure 7.7). There is often more than one (seldom more than three) point of retrograde filling in a limb.

There are further aids to the location of incompetent perforating veins. The point at which such a vein passes through the deep fascia is often tender and warm (a "hotspot"). There may be pigmentation over it. Incompetent perforating veins often bear a characteristic relation to varicose lesions. For example, a patch of eczema over the anterolateral aspect of the leg suggests incompetence of one of the anterior tibial perforating veins. Eczema or ulceration on the posterolateral aspect suggests incompetence in the peroneal or soleal perforating veins. A typical varicose ulcer above the medial malleolus is almost diagnostic of incompetence of a lower posterior tibial perforating vein, which may be beneath the base of the ulcer itself. The identification of incompetent perforating veins has been made much simpler with the advent of duplex scanning. Where this facility is available, it can be employed in the identification of sites of injection instead of the manual method.

Oedematous Legs

The method of examination described above is sometimes made impossible because of oedema of the lower limb. In this case, an elastic bandage and elastic stocking are applied from the base of the toes to above the biggest point of swelling. The patient is advised to walk as much as possible, to rest with the feet up two or three times a

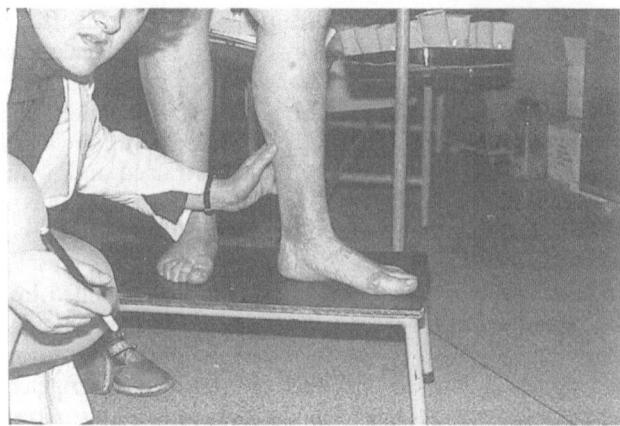

Figure 7.1 Patient standing ready to be marked. Also Plate VII.

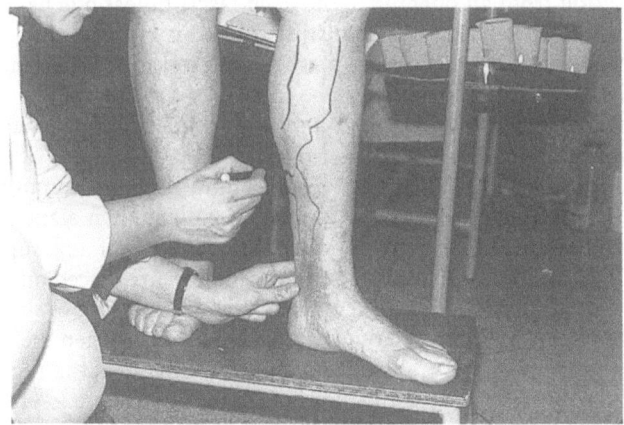

Figure 7.2 Dilated veins marked out following examination by inspection, palpation and percussion. Also Plate VIII.

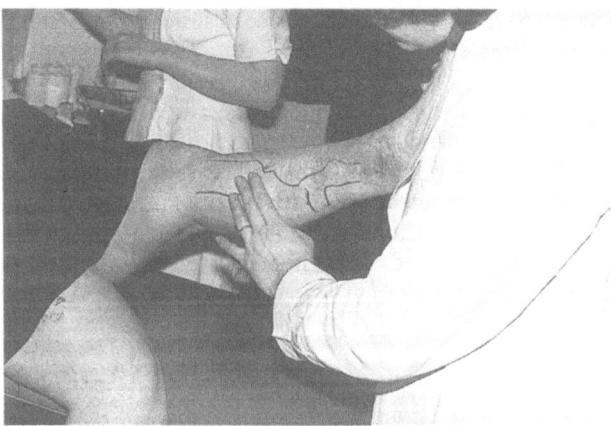

Figure 7.3 Patient lying down with the leg raised and the fascial orifices marked out, and the doctor palpating the raised leg. Also Plate VIII.

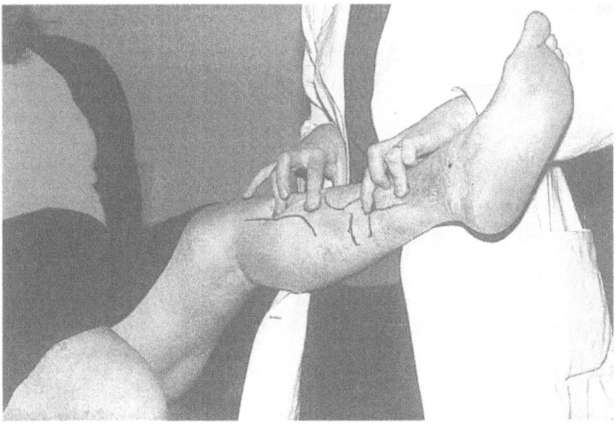

Figure 7.4 Doctor's fingers placed in fascial orifices with the patient's leg raised. Also Plate VIII.

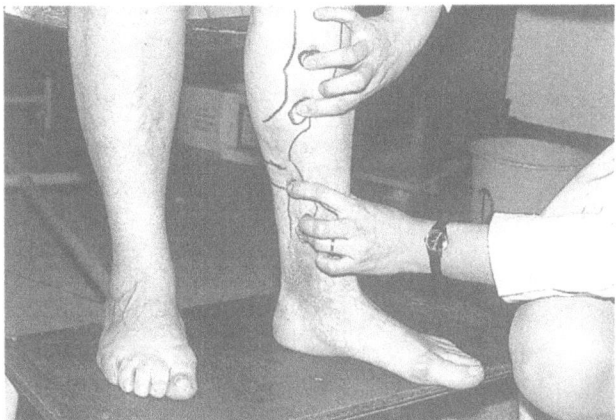

Figure 7.5 Filling of veins being controlled, with the patient standing, by finger pressure on fascial orifices. Also Plate IX.

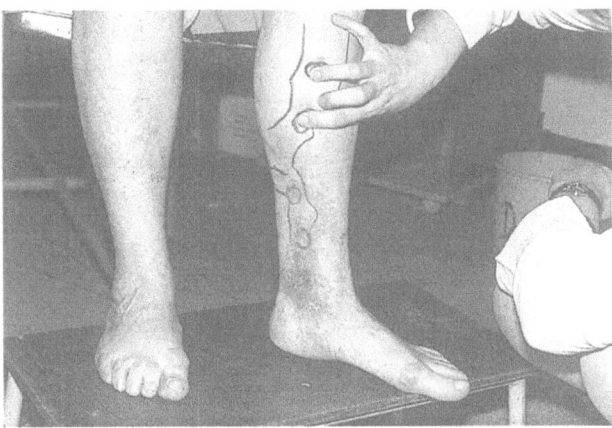

Figure 7.6 Removal of two fingers: veins do not fill. Also Plate IX.

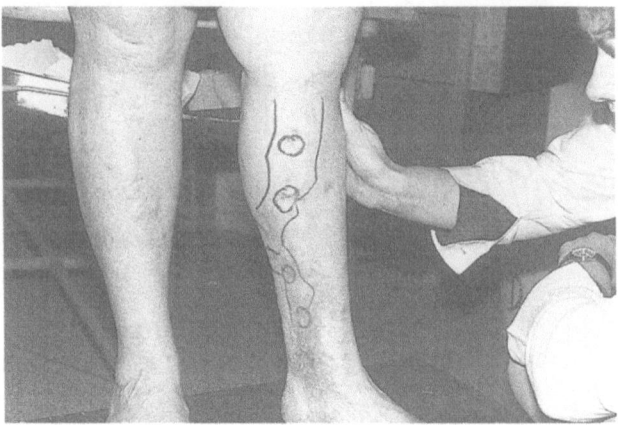

Figure 7.7 Removal of remaining fingers: veins fill. Also Plate IX.

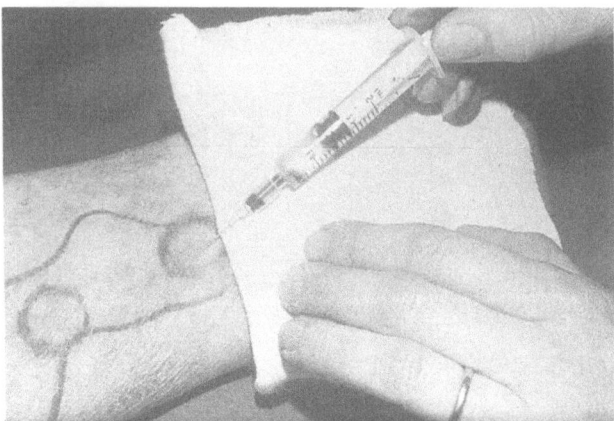

Figure 7.8 The needle is inserted into the vein while the patient sits on a couch. Also Plate X.

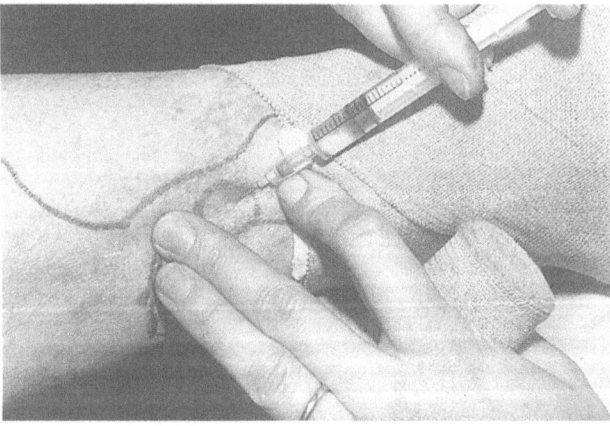

Figure 7.9 The leg is raised and the injection is given into a segment of vein isolated by firm compression by the ring and index fingers. Also Plate X.

day, and to raise the foot of the bed. After a month, the patient returns, having stayed in bed that day with the lower limbs elevated until it was time to leave home for the appointment with the doctor. On removing the stockings and bandages, the oedema is found to be greatly reduced, and it is now possible to detect the superficial veins and fascial orifices.

Sclerotherapy Technique

The patient sits upright on a couch, with the legs horizontal. The pressure of blood within the veins in this position is sufficient to make venepuncture possible. It is unnecessary for the patient to stand upright or for a tourniquet to be applied.

The most distal incompetent perforating vein should be injected first, followed by the next most distal, and so on until all the selected sites have been injected (Figure 7.8). This direction of progression is chosen so as to allow complete emptying of the veins for each injection; this is more difficult to achieve if there is already a tight bandage around the limb proximal to the injection site. However, if the distal perforating vein is injected first, the veins proximal to the site of injection may go into spasm, making injection of the more proximal sites impossible for several minutes. If two sites are at about the same level on the leg, they cannot both be injected at the same session. The vein that appears to have the more important relation to the complex of veins should therefore be injected first, with injection of the other vein postponed until the patient's second visit.

Injection

A 2-ml syringe containing 1 ml sodium tetradecyl and fitted with a 20-gauge disposable needle is used. Before injecting, it should be checked that the plunger of the syringe moves smoothly and freely. The skin at the site chosen for injection is cleansed, the needle is inserted, and a little blood is aspirated into the syringe to show that the tip of the needle is within the vein. About 0.1 ml of sclerosant is injected to clear the needle. The syringe is then held firmly against the leg, the patient lies back, and the leg is raised to empty the vein. The ring and index finger of the left hand (if the doctor is right-handed) are pressed on the vein above and below the needle, about 3 cm apart, in order to localise the effect of the injection (Figure 7.9). A total of 0.5–1 ml of sclerosant is injected into the isolated, almost empty segment of vein, and the needle is then removed. The sclerosant is retained in the isolated segment of the vein by the compressing fingers of the left hand for about 30 seconds.

The injection is normally painless. If the patient feels a stinging pain, this suggests that the sclerosant has been injected outside the vein and the injection should be stopped. Extravascular injection can usually be detected before it causes pain, because the resistance of the movement of the plunger of the syringe is greater than if it is intravascular. This difference can be detected only if the freedom of movement of the plunger has been tested before the injection is given.

Bandaging

A most important step in the technique is the bandaging. It cannot be overstressed that the best results are the results of the best bandaging. This part of the technique should be carried out by the doctor, and should not be delegated, except to somebody who is fully trained and known to be as competent. Three types of compression are used: bandages, rubber pads, and elastic stockings. All three are different in function and all are essential. The bandages used are of stiff cotton crepe and are 10 cm wide. The end of the bandage is secured with the middle finger or thumb of the left hand, and the bandage rolled around the leg, once above and once below the site of injection. The third turn covers the site of injection, and it is not until then that the fingers isolating the injected segment of vein are removed. A bevelled rubber pad is immediately placed over the injection site and bandaged firmly into position (Figure 7.10). The bevelling of these pads must extend to their edges in order to avoid the production of painful pressure marks on the legs. We have used pads of polyethylene foam, orthopaedic felt, and laminated gauze, as well as small dental gauze rolls, but these have all been rejected in favour of sorbo rubber. None of the other materials produced consistently satisfactory compression over the site of injection. Both hands are used simultaneously in bandaging; the right hand holds the bandage and wraps it round the limb, while the left hand, which is the more important, continuously palpates the bandage, assessing its firmness and tension. The correct result is achieved when the bandaged leg feels firm but the patient does not complain that the bandages feel too tight. It is the left hand that guides the right hand in the direction and tension with which the bandage is to be applied, by checking that the tension at the edges of the bandage is equal. If one edge of the bandage is tighter than the other, then the bandage will tend to slip. This method of bandaging is essential. If the bandages are applied in any other way, it cannot be claimed that compression sclerotherapy is being used.

Any other injections that may be necessary are given at the same session. Finally, further bandages are applied so that the limb is covered from the base of the toes up to just above the highest injection site. The ankle should be held in a neutral position between dorsiflexion and plantarflexion while being bandaged, and the knee should be slightly bent. A 10-cm^2 rubber pad is placed behind the knee and bandaged into position, as this prevents the bandages from rolling up at this site (Figure 7.11). Another piece of sponge rubber should protrude above the edge of the bandages over the LSV to prevent the sharp upper edge of the bandages traumatising the vein and causing ascending thrombophlebitis (Figure 7.12).

The pattern of bandaging is different in the various parts of the limb. The foot and ankle are bandaged with the figure-of-eight, the crossover taking place in front of the ankle. The spindle shape of the calf allows the bandage to spiral up and down the leg, forming a criss-cross pattern. The knee is bandaged with a figure-of-eight, the crossover taking place behind the knee over the rubber pad placed in the popliteal fossa. As the thigh is cone-shaped, it is necessary to make reverse turns at the upper limit of bandaging. If the thigh is fat, then the bandages have a strong tendency to roll down and become ineffective and dangerous by causing a constriction behind the limb and traumatising the superficial veins, causing ascending thrombophlebitis. It may therefore be necessary to secure the upper edge of the bandages with a turn of 10-cm elastic adhesive strapping. A full-length elastic stocking is fitted over the bandages (Figure 7.13). This stocking must be long enough to reach above the upper limits of the bandages and should be supported by a suspender belt. The stocking and suspender belt are worn day and night. The stocking has two functions: it applies compression to the whole limb, which is particularly valuable in holding the bandage in position after the disappearance of oedema, and, possibly more importantly, it prevents the bandages from becoming ruffled, especially at night. The rubber pad applies compression specifically to the site of injection, while the bandage provides

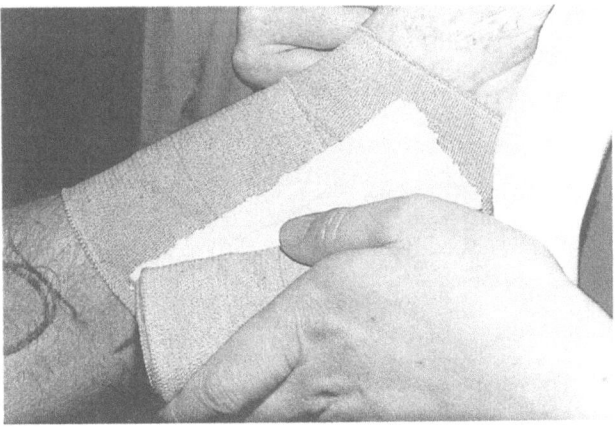

Figure 7.10 A sorbo pad is bandaged into position over the injection site. Also Plate X.

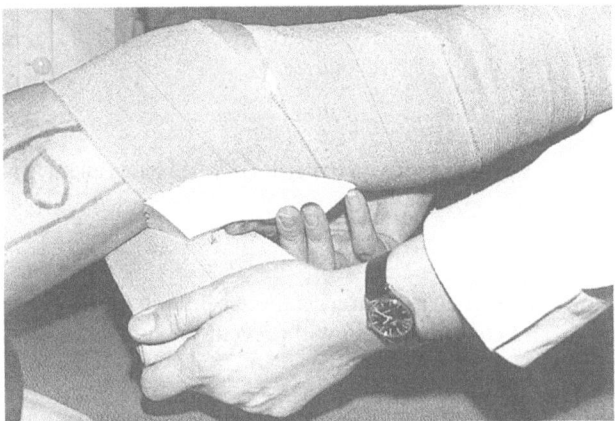

Figure 7.11 A rubber pad is placed behind the knee to prevent the bandages from rolling up and abrading the skin. Also Plate XI.

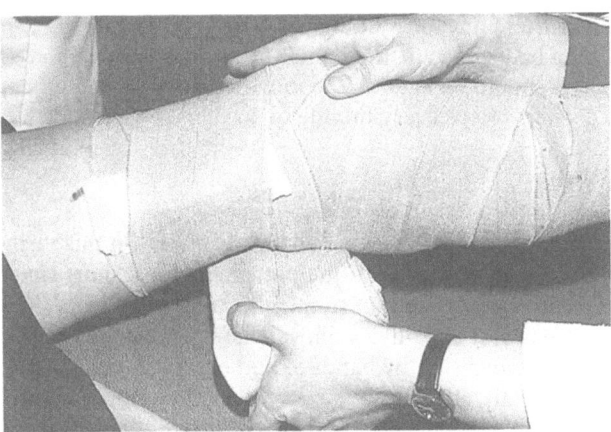

Figure 7.12 A rubber pad is left protruding above the upper edge of the bandages, preventing them from rolling down and forming a sharp ring, which would tend to traumatise the long saphenous vein and cause superficial thrombophlebitis. Also Plate XI.

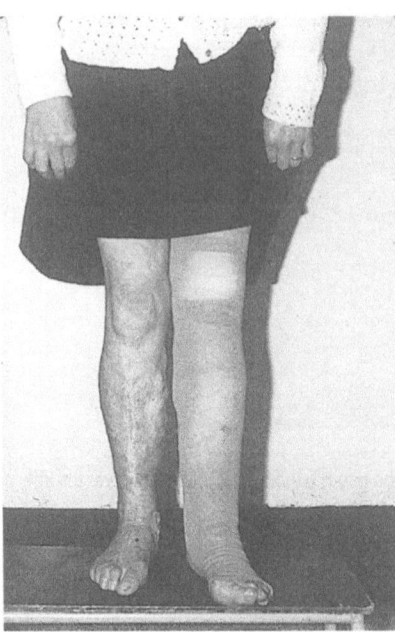

Figure 7.13 When bandaging is complete, an elastic stocking is applied and attached to a suspender belt. Also Plate XII.

what we describe as isometric pressure, i.e. there is little tendency for the bandage to increase in length, and consequently it will prevent the limb from swelling.

Walking

The patient is instructed not to remove either the stocking or the bandages until the next visit to the clinic, and to walk a total of three uninterrupted miles every day. The most important period for walking is the half-hour immediately after the injections, and the most important day for walking is the day of injection. It is emphasised that standing still is to be avoided. If the patient has to stay in one place for a length of time, then the feet should be kept on the move, either by going up and down on the toes or by taking a few steps every minute or so.

Subsequent Visits

The patient is seen one to two weeks after the injection. On this visit, it is quite safe to remove all bandages and to stand the patient up for a short time. The injection sites are examined, and the reactions to the injections are noted. The ideal result is a 5-cm segment of painless cord-like vein, which is only slightly tender to palpation. This lesion needs compression by bandage and elastic stocking until all tenderness has disappeared, usually after about six weeks. If the compression of the injection site has been insufficient, then a localised area of thrombophlebitis is found, equal in length to the distance between the localising fingers at injection. This area should be compressed firmly with bandages, rubber pad and elastic stocking until all tenderness has disappeared. This usually takes longer than six weeks. Occasionally, it is found that there has been no reaction to injection, in which case the injection is repeated, particular care being given to obtaining an empty segment of the injection site and to localising the sclerosant for a longer time. Very rarely, there is no reaction even after three injections at the same site. In such cases, we feel surgery is justified.

The veins are examined as before, and any further injections that are necessary are given. The limb is then bandaged again, the elastic stocking reapplied, and the patient instructed to continue the daily three miles of walking and to keep both the stocking and the bandages on all the time. The patient is seen at weekly or fortnightly intervals until no more injections are necessary. The next visit is arranged so that it will be at least six weeks after the last injection. At this visit, careful examination is made of the injection sites, particularly for residual tenderness. If an injected vein is still tender after six weeks of adequate compression, then very probably there is an undiagnosed incompetent perforating vein nearby. This should be searched for carefully and injected. Compression should not be removed until all tenderness has disappeared from the injection site, or for six weeks after the injection, whichever is longer. The patient is ready for discharge when all the injection sites have lost their tenderness, superficial veins have returned to normal size, and all the signs and symptoms in the limb have cleared up.

Patients frequently remark on a general improvement in their health and a feeling of wellbeing after their veins have been treated satisfactorily. Whether this is a specific result of improved venous return following treatment of the CVI, or whether it is due simply to the increased exercise that is part of the treatment, is uncertain. All patients should be followed up for at least five years. They should be seen three months after the course or treatment, and again at six months. Another visit one year after the course of treatment is important, as generally if recurrence is going to take place it will be within the first year. If recurrence occurs, then a further course of injection treatment can be given.

Complications of Treatment

Some patients suffer pain at the injection sites for a day or two following the injections. This is relieved by walking or by taking mild analgesics, such as aspirin, and is of no significance.

For several years, deliberate extravascular injections were given in the clinic in the belief that they produced a fibrous ring around the injected vein. In the light of experience and histological examination of biopsy specimens, it was discovered that this was not so. When the sclerosant does damage the skin, it may produce an area of necrosis. The slough later separates to leave an ulcer. These ulcers are usually painless if compression and ambulation have been adequate. A clean, dry dressing should be placed on the ulcer, and compression applied with bandages, rubber pad and elastic stocking. These ulcers heal rather slowly, and compression should be maintained until full epithelialisation is achieved.

An extravascular injection occasionally produces a circular patch of tissue damage that does not ulcerate. It is black in colour and painful. It should be treated by compression.

A patch of greenish-brown pigmentation sometimes appears over the injection site, especially if the reaction to the injection has been one of local thrombosis. This pigmentation later changes to brown and may persist.

Damage to a nerve by extravascular injection may cause pain or, if the damage is more severe, paraesthesia or numbness in the area of distribution of the nerve. This complication, which fortunately occurs very rarely, may take three to six months for recovery.

While it is probable that some of the injected sclerosant spills into the deep veins, in 16 000 patients treated in the clinic there has not been one in whom conclusive clinical signs of DVT were produced by an injection. The immediate ambulation following injection, by producing a rapid flow of blood along the deep veins, probably prevents any damaged area of intima from becoming a site for propagation of thrombus. The lytic activity of the vein wall and the circulating blood will also tend to reverse any thrombus formation.

No fatal case of pulmonary embolism has occurred in a patient undergoing compression sclerotherapy, nor are there any clinically proven cases of pulmonary embolism.

There have been about 15 cases of allergic reactions with hot stinging pain in the skin and an erythematous rash developing 30–90 minutes after injection. These cases were treated satisfactorily on subsequent visits by the administration of antihistamines before injection. Very rarely, a mild asthmatic attack has been caused. There have been about ten cases of mild anaphylaxis that required treatment with adrenaline. A severe reaction to an injection of sodium tetradecyl is a contraindication to further injections.

Specific Problems and their Treatment

Superficial Thrombophlebitis

Treatment of this condition may take two forms, depending on whether the patient is ambulant when first seen or whether the patient has been already been in bed for some time. In either case, careful examination is necessary to exclude the possibility of coexistent DVT.

If the patient is ambulant, then incompetent perforating veins in the vicinity or the lesion may be injected. A rubber pad is cut to the size and shape of the region of the thrombophlebitis and bandaged into position over the lesion. An elastic stocking is applied, and the patient is instructed to walk and to avoid standing. Anti-inflammatory analgesics are given to relieve the pain. If the lesion is fluctuant when first seen, then it may be aspirated, but squeezing blood clot out through an incision is unnecessary.

Post-thrombotic Leg

For certain diagnosis of previous DVT, duplex scanning or phlebography is essential. Following thrombosis of the deep vein, recanalisation to a major or minor degree is inevitable and usually takes place in a matter of six to eight weeks. However, the partially or totally recanalised vein is almost certainly valveless, or has damaged valves, and functioning with reduced efficiency.

Deep venous valve repair or transplantation is still experimental. Therefore, in the treatment of these cases it is most important to restore, as far as possible, the efficiency of the pumping mechanism in the foot, leg and thigh. That this approach is rational is shown by the fact that it is quite possible to tie a ligature on the iliac veins or even on the inferior vena cava and, if the pumping mechanisms are efficient, the venous return from the limb is adequate and the patient will suffer few if any symptoms in the affected limb. The idea that the varicose superficial and perforating veins form an alternative pathway for blood flow past the block in the deep veins is erroneous for the same reason.

These patients require treatment of their incompetent perforators more than patients with normal deep veins, because the damage to the valves in the deep veins reduces the efficiency of the pumping action and leaks through the incompetent perforating veins reduce it even further.

Clinically, these patients present with legs showing firm indurated oedema, thin glossy skin, and, frequently, ulceration. They often give a history of, or actually present with, a bursting sensation in the leg if they stand for any period of time. The thrombotic episode in the deep veins frequently follows pregnancy but sometimes it occurs after a fracture or after abdominal, pelvic or orthopaedic surgery. Treatment is carried out as described above, by locating and injecting the perforating veins that have incompetent valves. The damage to the valves in many cases is most probably due to the perforating veins having been involved in the thrombotic episode.

One can, with confidence, tell these patients that their symptoms will improve, that their swelling will decrease, and that their ulcers will heal. However, it should be made clear that the venous system cannot be restored to normality, and although complete symptomatic relief is to be expected it is wise to advise such patients to wear an elastic stocking during the daytime for the rest of their lives.

Varicose Eczema

The veins should be treated in the normal way, injecting through eczematous skin if necessary. Several layers of absorbent lint should be applied over the eczema, with compression preferably with plastic sponge rather than rubber. Antihistamines may be given if necessary to control itching. The patient should be encouraged to get plenty of exercise. If the eczema persists, then careful re-examination of the limb should be made for previously missed perforating veins. Persistent small patches may be treated with local corticoids. In almost all cases, the eczema clears when the venous disorder has been treated satisfactorily.

Varicose Ulcers

Many patients with non-varicose ulcers on their legs are referred to a clinic specialising in the treatment of venous disorders, and it is important to be on the lookout for them. Ulcers due to arterial insufficiency are common, and the possibility that an ulcer may be malignant should always be borne in mind, especially if the venous system is normal or diseased only mildly. Early biopsy is necessary in such cases. In the treatment of true varicose ulcers, the veins in the non-ulcerated areas are injected in the way described above. Dry dressings are applied to the ulcer and bandaged firmly in place, with a rubber pad over the ulcer to give extra pressure. The daily hour of walking should be carried out conscientiously, and the patient should sleep with the foot of the bed raised. Exercising the legs and ankles while lying in bed is also advisable. When the ulcer has healed, it is important to examine the site, since very frequently an incompetent perforating vein will be found there.

Telangectesia

Treatment of these is often sought for cosmetic reasons only and should be discouraged for the reasons already given. An exception is the "starburst" type of telangectesia, which is especially common in pregnancy and is often painful. There is frequently an incompetent perforating vein at the centre, and this should be injected as deeply as possible. The injection of sodium tetradecyl foam is often successful, but this may cause sloughing of the skin.

Combined Arterial and Venous Disease

Patients who suffer from both arterial inadequacy and chronic venous congestion of the lower limb may have their veins treated in the normal way, but great care should be taken that the compression does not reduce arterial flow below a safe level. Such patients are incapable of performing as much exercise as is usually advised, and this should be accepted. Exercise on a pedalling machine at home is a useful alternative. It has been found in many cases that treatment of the venous disorder also produces symptomatic relief of the arterial supply, and that this improvement is maintained.

Saphena Varices and Termination of the Long Saphenous Vein

Saphena varices will in all cases reduce, and in most cases disappear, following sclerosis of incompetent perforating veins in the calf and thigh. Compression at the saphenous opening after injection is impossible and therefore persistent saphena varices, if one insists that they must be treated, must be ligated. However, in 16 000 cases treated by injection sclerotherapy, it has never been necessary to perform a flush ligation at the saphenofemoral junction in order to obtain relief from symptoms. The disappearance of saphena varices and a thrill that follows restoration of normotension in the venous complex is accounted for by the recovery of function of the valves at the saphenous opening.

Treatment of Venous Insufficiency During Pregnancy

The technique of compression sclerotherapy was developed in the varicose vein clinic of the Rotunda Hospital, and a great part of the work has been carried out on pregnant women. While many workers hold that the definitive treatment of varicose veins during pregnancy is unnecessary and possibly meddlesome, our experience shows that not only is it valuable in producing symptomatic relief but also that it markedly reduces the incidence of venous complications during puerperium.

The appearance of varicose veins in pregnant patients suggests that varicosities reflect a generalised change in the patient's physiological condition, leading to dilation of lower-limb veins and the production of secondary valvular incompetence.

These changes appear to occur at a very early stage of pregnancy; some patients show marked venous dilation in the leg, with pain, even before the first missed menstrual period. These patients demonstrate that the leg-vein changes in pregnancy cannot be attributed to proximal venous obstruction by the gravid uterus, and that other factors must be involved, such as increased blood volume and flow or hormonal changes affecting the walls and valves of the vein.

The case against the treatment of varicose veins in pregnant women is based largely on the fact that a considerable degree of recovery occurs spontaneously following delivery. The significance of this observation is that it demonstrates unequivocally that varicose superficial veins are capable of returning to clinical normality in response to the physiological changes that occur postpartum. It must be stressed that full recovery does not occur in patients with primary valvular defect. The reserve capacity of the peripheral pump is often adequate to compensate for one or more leaking perforator veins. However, in patients with primary valvular defects, its capacity has been reduced permanently, and these women are prone to develop severe varicosities, with or without the burden of subsequent pregnancies. Furthermore, they bear an increased risk of thrombophlebitis and DVT during puerperium when the veins are recovering. The improvement that occurs at this stage is due to the restoration of competence in those valves that are affected secondarily by dilation of the veins. This would appear to affect the function in the same way as the application of an elastic stocking. Keane and Fegan in 1966 showed that this produced a diminution of the diameter of the superficial veins and a return of competence in the valves of those veins.

There are three principal reasons for treating varicose veins during pregnancy:

- Immediate relief of the distressing symptoms (cramps in the leg, tiredness, hot throbbing pain, swelling, eczema, ulceration) is provided.
- The ever-present danger of acute thrombophlebitis is minimised.
- In patients with a pre-existing mild degree of venous insufficiency, the vein walls may become damaged permanently because of the additional stress to which they are subjected during pregnancy, unless treated.

In pregnant patients, treatment of incompetent perforating veins will reduce the stress to which the superficial veins are subjected and facilitate the spontaneous return to normality.

The technique used in pregnant patients does not differ in any way from that described earlier. The diagnosis and localisation of the incompetent perforating veins are carried out in exactly the same manner in both pregnant and non-pregnant patients. These veins are injected, and compression is applied with bandages and elastic stockings. However, compression is maintained throughout the duration of the pregnancy, even in patients who no longer require further injections. In our clinic, treatment by injection continues throughout pregnancy without adverse effects. Patients are finally reviewed approximately six weeks after delivery, and any residual leaks are then dealt with. As in the case of non-pregnant patients, compression with an elastic stocking is maintained for two months after the bandages have been removed.

Vulval Varices

Varicosities of the labial veins develop frequently during pregnancy. They are particularly common in women who have undergone repeated pregnancies. While they are not strictly comparable with varicosities of the lower limb, much relief can be obtained by the use of a slightly modified technique of compression sclerotherapy. Opinion is divided with regard to the necessity for treating these varicosities.

McPheeters and Anderson in 1938 and Solomons in 1950 favoured active therapy during pregnancy, while Foote in 1960 stated that these veins are unsuitable for injection. We find that vulval varices are eminently suitable for compression sclerotherapy.

The case for the treatment of vulval varices can be argued on the same basis as that stated for the treatment of varices in the legs. Labial varices are a great source of discomfort and often cause considerable anxiety in pregnant patients. Many of them complain of extreme pressure in the vulva. Pruritus is common, and patients often suffer from a disturbing sensation of prolapse. The alleviation of these symptoms results in a considerable improvement of the patient's physical and psychological state throughout the pregnancy.

Extensive vulval varices, if untreated, may rupture during parturition, and fatal haemorrhage from vulval varices is not unknown.

The vulval veins are tributaries of the internal pudendal veins. They communicate with the vesical, vaginal and rectal venous plexuses, with the superficial external pudendal veins posteriorly, and with the superficial epigastric veins anteriorly. They become grouped together at the anterior and posterior aspects of the labia, and these points serve as the most suitable sites for injection.

Each injection consists of 1 ml 3% sodium tetradecyl mixed in the syringe with a little air so as to form a foam. This is then injected into the selected vein. When about 0.75 ml has been injected, the needle is withdrawn gently from the lumen of the vein, and the remainder of the injection is given immediately deep to and around the vein. While perivascular injection has been discarded from general use in the therapy of lower-limb varices, it has been found to be of value in the treatment of vulval veins and haemorrhoids.

Compression of the injection site is applied in the following manner: the patient wears four protective pads, which are held firmly over the vulva by a tight pair of two-way-stretch pants. Further injections are given as required at subsequent visits.

Results of Compression Sclerotherapy

There is no universally accepted standard by which the results of any method of treating CVI can be assessed and compared with the results obtained by other techniques. This is due in part to the wide variations that occur from one series to another in the acceptance of clinical features other than dilated veins and ulceration as being due to venous insufficiency. Thus, selection of cases presents an initial problem, which immediately affects the criteria by which the assessment is to be made. The early results following treatment are not of great value in patients treated by compression sclerotherapy, since patients are not discharged until they are considered to have been cured. The assessment of results after five or more years is complicated by the difficulty of distinguishing between recurrent and new varicosities. For simplicity, we consider as recurrences all varicosities that appear subsequent to treatment, and hence these patients are included as being unsatisfactory.

We studied 1171 patients attending for review out of a total of 1900 that had been treated over a ten-year period. They had all been treated by the same method, and they were all assessed by the overall results of treatment on individual signs and symptoms. In order to test whether the 1171 patients formed a representative sample of the 1900 patients asked to attend, the first 100 patients attending the clinic for each of three consecutive years were questioned in their homes. Some of these patients included those who attended the hospital on request; the others were those who had failed to keep their review appointment. The results of this questioning were so similar to the 1171 patients that the surveyed group was considered representative.

An independent worker interviewed the patients with regard to the following points:

- cramp in the legs at night;
- swelling of the legs or ankles;
- presence of large, distended veins on the leg;
- tiredness or heaviness of the legs;
- pain in the legs;
- ulceration of the legs;
- presence of a rash on the legs;
- presence of thrombophlebitis.

The history of the patient at the time of treatment was referred to at each interview in relation to these signs and symptoms.

The analysis resulted in 40 combination groups. The results were submitted to statistical testing to show the results of the treatment and the importance of two of the factors, compression and ambulation.

The patients were asked for an opinion about the general condition of their legs, and their replies were recorded as above. The patients were also asked whether they had worn their bandages continuously during treatment until told to remove them, whether they had found difficulty due to loosening or slipping in keeping the bandages on, and whether they had worn an elastic stocking over the bandages. Female patients were also asked whether they had been pregnant at the time of treatment, whether they had had any subsequent pregnancies, and, if so, how many.

Table 7.1 shows the results of treatment on all patients, both male and female, classified by signs and symptoms. The total for numbers treated (4519) differs from the total number of patients surveyed (1171), since most patients suffered from at least two of the signs or symptoms. The average cure rate for sign or symptom groups is statistically weighted by the number of patients in that particular group. The overall satisfactory result assessed by this method for 1171 patients, both mate and female, was 79.7%.

Table 7.1 Results of treatment on all patients (male and female) classified by symptoms and signs

Symptom or sign	Results of treatment		Patients treated (n)
	Satisfactory* (%)	Unsatisfactory** (%)	
Night cramp	83	17	685
Oedema	75	25	593
Large veins	81	19	974
Tiredness in legs	72	28	888
Pain in veins	79	21	594
Ulceration	91	9	340
Eczema	83	17	275
Phlebitis	89	11	170
All symptoms	79.7	20.3	4519

*Includes cured and improved; **includes no better and worse.

The name of the therapy, continuous compression sclerotherapy, implies the fundamental importance of adequate compression of the leg during treatment. The sample was divided into patients who maintained good compression and those who had bad compression. Those who kept on their bandages and elastic stockings continuously until told to remove them were classified as having had good compression. It was found that good compression produced a significant improvement in the overall score.

In general, the difference in the results of treatment between patients who had good rather than bad compression was greater than between good and bad walkers, although the overall difference was statistically significant in both cases. The individual signs and symptoms most affected by difference in compression were oedema, the presence of large, distended veins on the leg, and tiredness of the legs.

By these assessment standards, compression sclerotherapy gave an overall average satisfactory score of 79.7% of signs and symptoms for the whole group of patients, and 85.1% of signs and symptoms in those who maintained good compression and walked regularly. Altogether, 81.8% of the patients reviewed were satisfied with the results of treatment and considered themselves to be cured. Thus, it is clear that provided the technique is carried out carefully, compression sclerotherapy as practised in the Dublin Clinics produces a clinical result that compares favourably with any other method of treating CVI.

Advantages of Compression Sclerotherapy

In the large-scale treatment of any disease, the choice between different types of therapy yielding similar end results must be based upon factors such as ease of application, time involvement, and expense.

If the technique of compression sclerotherapy is followed rigidly, and satisfactory clinical results are obtained, then we believe that the adoption of this technique as the standard method of treating venous insufficiency offers considerable advantages to the individual patient, to the practitioner, and to the community at large. If the desirable clinical end results and satisfactory follow-up figures are not obtained, despite the fact that the practitioner feels they are using the technique correctly, then the practitioner would be well advised to discard this form of treatment. The resurrection of sclerotherapy as a treatment for varicose veins, unless adhered to rigidly as laid down by us, would be a retrograde step in the treatment of venous insufficiency.

Advantages to the Patient

In the treatment of approximately 16 000 cases by compression sclerotherapy, no deaths have occurred as a complication of the technique. Venous insufficiency is a condition in which direct fatal complications, such as exsanguination due to rupture of a varix, are exceptional, and therefore it is not permissible to advocate a method of treatment that carries even a small chance of mortality while an alternative method that reduces this risk is available. There is no doubt that compression sclerotherapy is safer for the patient than any other recognised therapeutic approach.

A small number of patients treated by compression sclerotherapy suffer from minor discomfort following the injections. The various causes of discomfort were discussed earlier. All of these result from errors in technique and, apart from the rare instances of sensitivity, can be avoided by proper attention to the placing of the injections, the localisation of the sclerosant, and the correct bandaging of the limb. Patients treated by compression sclerotherapy, including those with ulceration, are expected to continue their normal life during the course of their treatment. This is rarely possible with any other method of treatment as practised at present.

The routine treatment of patients as out-patients offers obvious advantages to them. The domestic upheaval, possible expense, and loss of earnings brought about by hospitalisation are avoided.

Patients treated by compression sclerotherapy do not have to obtain sick leave from their employment. It has been our policy to arrange for working patients to be seen in the evenings so that even short absences from work are unnecessary.

Frequently, surgical ligation or excision of varicose veins is marked by the development of unsightly scars at the sites of incision. While these may not appear to be an important factor to be considered in the choice of treatment, frequently they are a source of irritation and embarrassment to some patients, especially to those in whom the appearance of their legs may be important in their occupations.

The use of compression sclerotherapy enables a team of medical personnel to deal with much larger numbers of patients than they could reasonably care for by any other method, apart from palliative bandaging and dressing of ulcerated legs. Thus patients who otherwise would be relegated to a waiting list can expect to receive positive treatment quickly.

In the event of the development of further incompetent perforating veins or superficial varicosities in a patient being treated with compression sclerotherapy, all that will be required is a further course of injections. On the other hand, a patient being treated by operative methods must be subjected to the risks of a second anaesthetic and operation and the inconvenience of a further period of hospitalisation.

Advantages to the Doctor

As stated above, large numbers of patients can be dealt with quickly and efficiently by this method. Thus, it should be possible for any doctor to clear even a large list of patients waiting for treatment. However, a word of caution is necessary. Personnel who adopt compression sclerotherapy as a routine measure in the treatment of varicose veins frequently find that they are clearing not only their own waiting list but also those of several of their colleagues. There is a tendency among many practitioners to treat varicose veins either as a nuisance or with studied neglect, and naturally patients tend to gravitate towards those who offer them immediate and positive therapy.

Most general hospitals in the UK and Ireland have an ever-present problem in providing hospital beds for those for whom hospitalisation is essential. The treatment as out-patients of patients with varicose veins immediately removes a very substantial burden from the hospital bed situation.

By compression sclerotherapy, patients can be treated more rapidly than by any other technique. As a result, time is spared, which can be employed usefully for other purposes.

Even if the results of compression sclerotherapy were to compare only reasonably with those of other techniques, the advantages listed above would strongly support the case for its general adoption. However, we believe that properly practised compression sclerotherapy can be expected to produce better end results, in terms of relief of symptoms as well as disappearance of obvious varicosities, than those generally obtained by surgery.

Advantages to the Community

These are, in the main, economic. The use of compression sclerotherapy saves doctors' time, saves nurses' time, saves hospital beds and their attendant expenses, reduces loss of earnings due to absence from work, does not cause dislocation of industry due to absence of key operators, and does not cause disruption of home life.

In any large community, economic considerations are necessarily a major factor in the provision of health services. In scientific disciplines other than medicine, a constant search continues for techniques that will reduce the economic burden on the community. Venous insufficiency is such a common ailment that if it were possible to discontinue the hospitalisation of these patients, then the gain to the community would be measurable in millions of pounds.

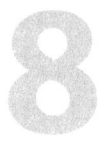

Review of the Literature

T.R. Cheatle

Despite the fact that the history of sclerotherapy can be traced back at least 150 years, the place of the technique in the treatment of venous disease remains unclear. The invention of the hypodermic syringe in the mid-nineteenth century led to several reports of attempted obliteration of varicosities by injection. Cassaignac seems to have been the first in print, in 1855, using a solution of ferric perchloride. Throughout the second half of the nineteenth century, case reports and small series were published, using different sclerosant solutions, with a common theme of unpleasant and frequent complications. Despite this, interest in the technique as an alternative to operation continued, perhaps because of the risks associated with surgery at the time. Linser first described the combination of injection treatment with compression by bandages in 1916. In their treatment of the subject, Browse and colleagues called Linser "probably the father of modern compression sclerotherapy". However, Linser's use of hypertonic saline led to problems of pain and ulceration when extravasation occurred.

Modern sclerotherapy may be thought to date from the use of sodium tetradecyl sulphate, described by Tournay in 1931. This substance is a detergent, being the salt of an alkaline metal and a long-chain fatty acid. It is used in different concentrations, from 0.5% to 3%, depending on the size of the vessel being injected. Its action is to cause an intense chemical phlebitis leading to obliteration of the vein, an obliteration made more effective by firm compression.

Reports of personal series of patients treated by sclerotherapy were numerous in the 1950s and 1960s and were generally very positive. Although typified by relatively short follow-up periods and occasionally rather broad definitions of what constitutes good results, it became clear from these papers that sclerotherapy was an effective technique in many patients. Quantification of the success rate of sclerotherapy has always been difficult, depending as it usually does on such "soft" data as reports of patient satisfaction and the surgeon's opinion regarding the degree of cosmetic improvement.

Surveying the literature on venous sclerotherapy shows that the number of key papers is quite small. We have included as key papers those that represent scientific attempts to answer important questions about the technique, or those that have been exceptionally influential.

Key Papers in the Literature of Venous Sclerotherapy[*]

Karl Sigg

Karl Sigg (1952) worked in the Women's Hospital, Basle, Switzerland, but his long and frequently quoted paper was stimulated by a visit to the USA. While there, he was surprised to find a strong prejudice in favour of surgery as opposed to sclerotherapy for varicose veins. This stemmed from the perception that sclerotherapy took a long time, was associated with a high rate of recurrence, and had some unpleasant complications. Although he was writing 50 years ago, it would be true to say that these opinions are still held by many vascular surgeons.

He addressed these points with the following arguments. Although sclerotherapy may take several visits to achieve the desired result, it leads to much less time off work than does surgery. For fee-paying patients, it is also much cheaper and thus may encourage patients to seek care earlier, leading to better results.

As regards recurrences, Sigg accepts that they occur, but he opines that the frequency is no greater than with surgery "if sclerotherapy is carried out properly". By this, he meant that the leg should be horizontal at the time of injection, that intravenous haematomas should be removed under local anaesthetic, that compression bandaging should be used, and that the patient should be reviewed regularly.

The complications following surgery for varicose veins were, at the time, bedevilled by the spectre of DVT and pulmonary embolism, which occurred in nearly 1% of cases. This represented a strong pressure to pursue safer treatments, such as sclerotherapy, where death from pulmonary embolism was almost unheard of. Smith and Johnson (1948) quote one death in a series of 11 700 cases. Severe anaphylactic reactions, although described, are also rare. The principal complications of the technique – staining, ulceration due to extravasation, superficial thrombophlebitis – are uncomfortable rather than life-threatening and can be minimised by expert technique.

Sigg goes on to describe the technique that he believes should be used for injection sclerotherapy. He emphasises that the leg should be horizontal. He makes the interesting suggestion that hydrostatic pressure might make sclerosant seep back along the outside of the needle and cause skin necrosis if the patient is standing. He stresses that the needle should not be too small (in order to allow a better "feel" of when one is inside or outside a vein). Injection should be by the air-block technique. He lays great importance on the need for compression and early ambulation.

The final half of Sigg's paper is not relevant to sclerotherapy, dealing as it does with the problems of venous ulceration and effective compression bandaging.

Sigg is one of the major figures in the development of compression sclerotherapy. The technique of inserting the needle with the patient in the standing position but injecting with the leg horizontal is attributed to him. He also recommended starting sclerotherapy in the most distal varices as opposed to Tournay, who had recommended starting at the most proximal point of reflux. In addition, Sigg was among the first to stress the desirability of graduated compression rather than uniform compression. For these innovations as much as for his enthusiastic and detailed publications, he is remembered as one of the founders of modern sclerotherapy.

---

[*]For full references please see Further Reading.

W.G. Fegan

George Fegan's name has become synonymous with the use of sclerotherapy in many parts of the world. In two early papers (Fegan, 1960; Fegan, 1963), he describes his technique in detail and his experiences of treating 13 352 patients. In the first paper, dealing especially with his experience of treating pregnant women at the Rotunda Hospital in Dublin, he makes the remark that the aim of his treatment is "to concentrate rather on restoring the efficiency of the [calf muscle] pump than on obliterating apparent superficial varices". He describes his injection method in detail in Chapter 7 of this book. Fegan makes the point strongly that the aim of sclerotherapy is not to cause thrombosis in a varix, but rather to cause an obliterative fibrosis. Histological evidence is adduced to show the recanalisation that occurs when a vein has been merely thrombosed compared with the absence of the same when fibrous obliteration has been achieved.

This obliteration, as Fegan describes in the second paper, is obtained by immediate and continuous compression sustained for six weeks. Great importance is laid on the technique of bandaging.

An unselected group of 760 patients was studied for recurrence over a six-year period and satisfactory results were found in 84.6%, based on both subjective and objective assessment.

Fegan's papers are essentially descriptive and do not purport to be trials. Clearly, as his results show, he was an expert and dedicated exponent of the method he developed. His emphasis on using an "empty vein" technique, the importance he placed on controlling points of reflux (especially the Hunterian perforator above the femoral condyle) rather than simply injecting varices at random, and his bandaging technique have all formed the basis of most sclerotherapy done in many parts of the world today.

John T. Hobbs

Hobbs (1974) provided one of the first attempts to compare in a scientific way the outcome of the two techniques. In the key part of his paper, 500 patients with varicose veins were randomised to either surgical or injection treatment. The patients were photographed and classified by severity before treatment. However, no data are given as to the pathophysiology in these patients, e.g. long or short saphenous incompetence. Injection treatment was performed using Hobbs' own method, which involves inserting the needle and injecting with the patient flat. (This differs from Fegan's method, where the patient has the needles placed while sitting with their legs hanging over the side of a couch, and is then asked to lie flat for the injection of sclerosant.) Sodium tetradecyl sulphate 3% was used. An average of 11.4 injections per leg were given, although we are not told how many sessions were required. The legs were bandaged for six weeks. A minor flaw in the study was that those patients allocated to surgery were treated by a number of different surgeons, presumably of differing experience and ability, although Hobbs states that "most" of the operations were done by him. The patients were seen and reassessed at six-monthly intervals for up to six years, and classified as cured, improved or failed, according to the least favourable view of either patient or surgeon.

Hobbs found that after one year, patients treated by sclerotherapy had a better result than those operated upon. However, over subsequent years, this difference disappeared and was reversed due to increasing numbers of recurrences seen in the injection group. This was despite intermittent extra injection treatments given to patients in the sclerotherapy group. By six years, approximately 20% of the surgical group were classified as failures compared with almost 70% of the sclerotherapy group. Hobbs concluded that patients with definite saphenofemoral or popliteal reflux were best served by surgery while those without should receive sclerotherapy, a view that would be accepted widely by many vascular surgeons practising today.

A.D.B. Chant, H.O. Jones and J.M. Weddell
S.A.A. Beresford, A.D.B. Chant, H.O. Jones, D. Piachaud and J.M. Weddell

Chant et al. (1972) and Beresford et al. (1978) give the results of another randomised controlled trial in which 115 patients were treated with compression sclerotherapy and 100 were treated by surgery. Again, we do not know how many had long or short saphenous incompetence, or neither. Ninety patients were excluded from the trial because they had recurrent or trivial veins, or had medical or social contraindications, or because they expressed a strong preference for one form of treatment.

Surgical treatment consisted of saphenofemoral or saphenopopliteal ligation, stripping of the LSV or SSV, and ligation of any clinically detected perforators. Injection sclerotherapy was performed using Fegan's method (see Chapter 7). Information concerning the number of injections and the number of sessions used was not given.

The patients were followed up at six months and at yearly intervals thereafter. Chant et al. (1972) wrote their paper when 93% of patients had achieved a three-year follow-up. Patients were classified depending on their requirement for further treatment, be it surgery, sclerotherapy or stockings. Including those who declined any treatment after randomisation, the authors found that 25% in the surgical group had required further treatment compared with 27% in the group treated by compression sclerotherapy. On these results, the authors concluded that the two treatments were equivalent in their effect. They also made the point that sclerotherapy was often more acceptable to women with children, as it avoided a disruptive hospital admission, even if several out-patient visits were required.

In the paper by Beresford et al. (1978), the same patients were reviewed, having now been followed up for a minimum of five years. At this stage, 40% of those initially treated by sclerotherapy had required some form of retreatment, compared with 24.2% of those treated surgically. Interestingly, the authors found that difference was principally in older patients; in those patients younger than 35 years, the two treatments remained equivalent. The results of this paper indicated a long-term advantage to surgical treatment, although the scale of the difference in results is quite small.

John Seddon

A total of 201 patients with demonstrable incompetence of the saphenous systems and/or ulceration due to perforator incompetence were studied by Seddon (1973). They were divided (presumably randomly, although the paper does not say this) to receive either surgical treatment (saphenofemoral disconnection with stripping of the LSV and perforator ligation) or sclerotherapy by Fegan's method. Patients undergoing sclerotherapy were reviewed every three weeks until treatment was deemed complete; the average number of injections was not given. Post-treatment compression was applied using bandages, although the duration is not stated.

Follow-up was between 12 and 18 months in all cases. Twenty-nine of the 149 (19%) limbs treated by sclerotherapy did not respond to treatment (three limbs) or had residual (19 limbs) or recurrent (seven limbs) veins at follow-up. This compares with 25 of 125 (20%) limbs treated surgically. Two of the 15 patients with ulcers in the sclerotherapy group suffered ulcer recurrence, compared with none of the five treated surgically. A small number of minor complications occurred in both groups.

The author concludes that the outcome of the two treatment methods is approximately the same. This agrees with the findings of other studies for the follow-up period described, but whether that equivalence would have been maintained over a longer period is a moot point; the studies of Hobbs (1974), Chant et al. (1972) and Beresford (1978), described above, would suggest not.

F.S.A. Doran and Mary White

Motivated largely by the length of time patients were staying in hospital following varicose vein surgery (10.5 days), Doran and White (1975) designed this trial to compare surgical treatment with sclerotherapy. A total of 502 limbs in 331 patients with primary uncomplicated varicose veins were randomised (by year of birth) to receive either sclerotherapy by Fegan's method (280 limbs) or conventional surgery (222 limbs). No details of exactly what types of operations were performed are given. In the sclerotherapy group, 64.6% of patients had between one and five visits, with no more than four injections being given at a time; 23.8% had between six and ten visits; and 11.6% had over ten visits. Outcome was measured at one and two years simply by ascertaining whether patients had required further treatment (i.e. injections). Subjective or objective evaluation of the limbs is not described.

At the end of one year, 24.2% of limbs in the sclerotherapy group had required further treatment, compared with 44.8% in the surgical group. After an additional year's follow-up, another 21.3% in the injection group and 16.4% in the surgical group had received further treatment, although, as the authors admit, the high dropout rate by this stage (about one-third) made these results of uncertain significance.

The authors conclude "the initial response of varicose veins is better if Fegan's method is used than if they are operated upon".

This is the only randomised trial to come down in favour of sclerotherapy over surgical treatment. Unfortunately, there appear to be too many flaws in the study to warrant its rather grand title. The follow-up period is too short: other studies agree that after one year, results of the two forms of treatment may be similar but that the recurrence rate rises in the injection group therafter. The requirement of almost half the surgically treated group to have injection sclerotherapy within a year of operation is troubling. As mentioned, we do not know what operations were carried out, but this figure suggests that the surgeons involved may have been less than assiduous in their performance of multiple avulsions. The method of deciding whether treatment has failed seems intrinsically unfair: patients receiving sclerotherapy can go on doing so at weekly intervals for an indefinite period until the clinician is satisfied, whereas surgical patients needing, perhaps, just one or two postoperative injections are classed as treatment failures.

The paper confirms that skilled sclerotherapy is an effective treatment for varicose veins in the short to medium term, but it cannot be said to have shown it to be a superior treatment to surgery.

B.H. Jakobsen

The work by Jakobsen (1979) is one of the key papers on the subject by being one of the very few studies to compare directly surgical and sclerotherapeutic treatment. However, the work suffers in its subjective method of classification and assessment. Through no fault of its author, the paper was written a few years before Doppler examination and duplex ultrasound became standard objective methods of assessment of venous abnormality.

A total of 516 patients who presented with saphenous varices were stratified to one of three treatment groups. It is unclear whether this was a randomisation. The three groups comprised 161 patients who had "radical surgery" – junctional ligation with excision of the LSV and/or SSV – 165 patients who had junctional ligation under local anaesthetic combined with sclerotherapy, and 157 patients who had sclerotherapy alone (Sigg's method). No information is given concerning the number of treatment sessions or the number of injections per session in the sclerotherapy group.

Patients were followed up at three months and at three years. Their outcome was classified both objectively and subjectively. Results for all treatments were, broadly speaking, very good at three months, but differences were demonstrated at the three-year follow-up. By objective evaluation, 89.8% of patients undergoing radical surgery had satisfactory results, as had 65.2% in the local surgery + sclerotherapy group. Only 36.6% of those having sclerotherapy alone were classified as objectively satisfactory at three years. Interestingly, the patients' subjective evaluations of their outcome showed less striking differences, with 93%, 84.8% and 70.5%, respectively, reporting that they were satisfied with the results at three years. The authors conclude that "radical surgery" is the best treatment for varicose veins.

P. Reddy, J. Wickers, T. Terry, P. Lamont, J. Moller and J.A. Dormandy

Fegan originally proposed six weeks as being the ideal period of compression following injection sclerotherapy. Patients often find this uncomfortable and inconvenient, so Reddy et al. (1986) performed two trials of one versus three weeks' compression and three versus six weeks' compression. All patients were without clinical evidence of saphenofemoral or saphenopopliteal incompetence. Immediately after the injections had been performed, patients were allocated to receive either one or three weeks' (trial 1, 145 legs) or three or six weeks' (trial 2, 169 legs) compression. Thereafter, a doctor unaware of the compression period evaluated the patients at three months and then at yearly intervals. The doctor evaluated phlebitis, pigmentation, induration, and the presence or absence of varicosities. The patients also assessed themselves using a questionnaire.

The trial comparing one versus three weeks' compression showed no difference between the groups at three months. However, by two years, there was a statistically significant difference, both in terms of the patients' self-assessment and in the independent examination, in favour of a three-week compression period.

The trial comparing three versus six weeks' compression had different results. After three months, the groups demonstrated no difference in outcome, either subjectively or objectively. This remained the case throughout the full six-year follow-up.

These authors have demonstrated clearly that a three-week period of compression after sclerotherapy is better than one week and as good as six weeks. However, one must remember that these are patients with reticular veins only, and one would have to be cautious about extrapolating this to patients who did have long or short saphenous incompetence.

J.R. Pfeifer and G.D. Hawtof

Some may argue against the work of Pfeifer and Hawtof (1989) being described as a key paper, as it is essentially anecdotal, without proper scientific descriptions of outcome measurements. However, it serves to highlight the fact that most surgeons, whatever their opinion of injection sclerotherapy for varicose veins, accept that it is the treatment of choice for telangiectasia.

One hundred and twenty-one patients were treated by CO_2 sclerotherapy over a three-year period. A Cavitron CO_2 laser was used to perform multiple dot entries along the course of the telangiectasia. The leg was then bandaged for three weeks. At the end of this period, it was found that prominent scarring was always present. These scars generally faded by the end of three months. Complications of the procedure included a high recurrence rate, pain at the time of the procedure, and occasional pigmentation. The most serious problem was persistent scarring, which, as the procedure in these patients was for purely cosmetic purposes, led to many patients rejecting the technique. The authors claim a 69% rate of "good to excellent" results, although how this figure is arrived at is not made clear. "Most patients" found scar formation "disturbing".

Because of dissatisfaction with this technique, the authors moved towards injection sclerotherapy, using hypertonic saline and a three-week compression period. A total of 598 patients were treated over a seven-year period. An average of three treatments was given per patient, with an average of 15 injections per treatment. Out of a total of 28 253 injections, six resulted in ulceration due to extravasation. The authors claim a 90% patient satisfaction rate, but details are not given.

Clearly this is not a trial of one treatment against the other, and essentially it is anecdotal. Nevertheless, in view of the large numbers of patients involved, the paper carries some weight in supporting compression sclerotherapy as a superior treatment for telangiectasia compared with laser treatment.

E. Einarsson, B. Eklof and P. Neglen

At the time of writing, the paper by Einarsson et al. (1993) is the most recently published of the very few randomised trials comparing surgery with sclerotherapy. A total of 164 patients with symptomatic primary varicosities were randomised to either operative treatment or compression sclerotherapy. Patients were assessed clinically and by foot volumetry before treatment. Eighty patients underwent surgery and 84 had compression sclerotherapy. Patients were well matched for age, sex, and pattern of venous disease. The type of surgery was determined by the clinical diagnosis, e.g. long or short saphenous incompetence, and the presence or absence of perforating vein incompetence. Sclerotherapy was performed by Hobbs' modification of Fegan's technique. An average of five injections per patient was given over one, two or three sessions. Patients in both groups had four to six weeks of post-treatment compression.

Patients were followed up at six months, one year, three years and five years. They were assessed by clinical inspection, subjective opinion of the patient, and foot volumetry. Follow-up compliance was reasonably good, with 78% (compression sclerotherapy) and 76% (surgery) attending for the full five-year follow-up.

At one year, 97% of surgical patients and 82% of compression sclerotherapy patients considered themselves cured or improved. The physician's assessment was 93% and 80%, respectively. The results in the compression sclerotherapy group fell away over the following four years. By five years, 95% of surgical patients still considered themselves cured or better, compared with only 45% in the compression sclerotherapy group; objective assessment gave figures of 90% and 26%, respectively. The foot volumetry results, measuring expelled volume (a measure of calf muscle function) and refilling flow (a measure of reflux), gave broadly similar results: 10% of operated patients had problems with sural or saphenous nerve damage, while 22% of compression sclerotherapy patients had had problems with superficial thrombophlebitis. Most of this was minor, but five patients required surgery because of phlebitis in the LSV and were thus classed as failures.

This seems to have been a well-conducted trial, the results of which support those of Hobbs (1974) and Jakobsen (1979). The trial started just before duplex scanning became generally available, but foot volumetry is a valid method for assessing calf muscle function and refilling times, and has been show to correlate well with direct venous pressure measurements. However, the average number of injections (five) given to patients in the sclerotherapy arm of the trial seems remarkably small, leading to the inevitable question as to whether more assiduous treatment in this group might not have led to a better outcome. In addition, the high rate of post-injection superficial thrombophlebitis suggests that the empty-vein technique required by Fegan may not always have been achieved.

U. Baccaglini, G. Spreafico, C. Castoro and P. Sorrentino

The paper by Baccaglini et al. (1997) summarises the proceedings of three consensus conferences held (twice) in Padua and Venice in 1994 and 1995. Thirty-one participants (all but one European) and eight further participants (six from outside Europe) met to answer the question: is sclerotherapy effective and, if so, under what circumstances? Participants and contributors were acknowledged experts, invited by nomination from national phlebological societies. It was felt that personal experience was of greater importance in this area than in many other areas in medicine, since the low scientific standard of many phlebological publications made an evidence-based approach difficult. A questionnaire was sent to over 1000 phlebologists worldwide in order to reveal current practice in the field of sclerotherapy.

The consensus statement discussed and reached conclusions in the following areas: indications, pretreatment assessment, techniques, results and training.

Indications

It was agreed that sclerotherapy is the treatment of choice for small varicose veins. Unfortunately, the term "small" is not defined, but it includes telangiectasia and reticular veins.

For larger veins not arising from an incompetent saphenous trunk, it was agreed that sclerotherapy was an "adequate" treatment, although there appears to have been some dissent about its role in treating incompetent perforating veins.

No consensus could be reached on whether varicosities arising from an incompetent LSV should be treated by sclerotherapy. It was agreed that veins arising from an incompetent short saphenous system could be treated by either surgery or sclerotherapy, but it was felt that there was inadequate evidence in the literature to give any recommendations on this point.

Agreement was reached that the following circumstances constituted absolute contraindications to the use of sclerotherapy: allergy to the sclerosing agent, severe systemic disease, recent DVT, infection, inability to walk, and severe arterial disease.

Pretreatment Assessment

Clinical findings, handheld Doppler, duplex scanning, plethysmography and PPG were all discussed, but no agreement could be reached on which, apart from clinical assessment, were necessary before sclerotherapy was commenced. It was agreed that for research studies, objective data from duplex scanning and some form of plethysmography must be gathered if the study is to be meaningful. However, it was also recognised that by the nature of the disease, a "good result" may be attainable in the absence of any objective measure of haemodynamic improvement.

Techniques

The participants suggested that rigid adherence to any of the three main techniques (Tournay's, Sigg's, Fegan's) should be abandoned and that "the choice of technical elements from the various schools be left to the discretion of each physician". They stress that the clinician should have a standardised technique, whatever its details.

It was agreed, not very surprisingly, that small varicose veins should be injected using small needles. Pre-injection aspiration is recommended where possible, although obviously not for telangiectasia. It was agreed that small veins should be injected with the leg horizontal.

Very little consensus was achieved in deciding the best way to inject large varicose veins. It was recommended that one of four solutions be used when treating large veins: iodine, sodium tetradecyl sulphate, polidoconol or sodium salicylate. It was agreed that post-procedure compression is mandatory if one is using a bottom-up technique (Sigg's or Fegan's) but not if one uses the top-down technique (Tournay's). The type and duration of compression could not be agreed on. Echosclerotherapy was discussed and recommended for use in recurrent, short saphenous, anterior saphenous, and perforating veins, and also in obese patients.

Results

The participants highlighted the shortcomings in the small number of randomised controlled studies that have been reported. The discrepancies between the excellent results of personal series and those of randomised trials are also pointed out. The participants agreed that it was impossible to say whether sclerotherapy prevented complications of varicose veins. In future studies, the following outcome measures were suggested: prevention and treatment of complications, patient satisfaction, reattendance, lack of effect, side effects, recurrence of varicose veins, and cost. An ideal study was proposed, which would have the following characteristics:

- Prospective, randomised, controlled.
- Homogeneous patient sample, e.g. all LSV varicosities. Pre-procedure investigation would be mandatory to ensure this.

- Standardised sclerotherapy technique.
- All complications and side effects of treatment to be recorded.
- Independent assessment of objective criteria when measuring outcome.
- At least five years' follow-up, with full details of all subsequent treatment.

Training

The unsystematic way in which sclerotherapy is taught was disparaged, and recommendations were made regarding the institution of recognised centres of training. Trainees should be examined and awarded a certificate when deemed competent in the technique.

This paper is a thorough and honest attempt to reach clear recommendations about the practice of sclerotherapy in venous disease. Unfortunately, perhaps even inevitably, the consensus recommendations are so unexceptional as to be anodyne. This may be due to the large number of participants, but more importantly it reflects the poor quality of the literature available, which the authors recognise. It is disappointing that instead of making suggestions about how to find out which sclerotherapy technique works best, the authors make the rather bland suggestion that it is left to individual clinicians to use the method they like best. The most useful part of the document is the outline of the ideal study in examining the efficacy of sclerotherapy, which should act as a model for future investigators

R.B. Galland, T.R. Magee and M.H. Lewis

The premise of Galland et al. (1998) is that sclerotherapy, although having been used widely for decades, has not become an integral part of every surgeon's practice. Three hundred and fifty members of the Vascular Surgical Society of Great Britain and Ireland were contacted by post and asked about the place of venous sclerotherapy in their practice. They were also asked whether their use of the technique was increasing or decreasing with time. A total of 218 (62%) replied: 18.3% claimed to never use sclerotherapy; only 4.6% used it when the patient was known to have proximal junctional incompetence, whereas 69.7% used it when such incompetence was absent; 77% used the method to treat residual varices left behind after operation; and 64.7% used it to treat recurrent varices without junctional incompetence.

The median compression time was less than that usually recommended by the inventors of the technique. The median time after sclerotherapy for varicose veins was two weeks, while after sclerotherapy for telangiectasia it was only four days.

The trend was for surgeons to use sclerotherapy less frequently for varicose veins than before, but more often for telangiectasia.

One important point emerging from this study was that only 33% of respondents used sclerotherapy and had a specialised varicose vein clinic. Clearly, this limits the scope for training junior surgeons. Lack of proper training may lead to poor technique, and this may contribute to what some would see as an ongoing underuse of the method.

Conclusions

The papers described above give a snapshot of the current feeling about the use of sclerotherapy. The majority of trials that compare surgery with sclerotherapy for primary varicose veins indicate that the results are similar over the medium term, but that in the long term surgery is more durable, with fewer recurrences. Most vascular surgeons agree that sclerotherapy is the treatment of choice for thread veins, and use the technique for these and for residual or recurrent veins after definitive surgery.

One problem that occurs in comparing surgery with sclerotherapy is that the latter, especially, is dependent on the degree of skill and commitment with which it is applied. Whereas stripping the LSV is basically an all-or-nothing procedure, the outcome of which is likely to be much the same whether it is done smoothly or clumsily (within limits), the same cannot be said of injection treatment. Inexpertly performed sclerotherapy is likely to lead to very poor results and many complications. Thus, committed advocates of the technique, who spend a great deal of time and concentration in using the method, are likely to get better results than those who view it as an inferior treatment and use it reluctantly. The argument that papers that report poor outcomes following sclerotherapy do so because the injections were done improperly or insufficiently, or with inadequate compression, is always going to be difficult to counter, and it may well, of course, have some truth in it.

Conclusions

S.K. Shami and T.R. Cheatle

Enthusiasm for sclerotherapy varies from one country to another, and from one decade to another. Although it is performed widely in the USA and mainland Europe, the technique is relatively unpopular in Britain, where surgery is the usual treatment for varicose veins. It is our impression that this may be changing. Whether this is out of interest in new techniques, such as ultrasound-guided sclerotherapy, or new materials, such as sclerosant foam, or whether it is for the more mundane reason that the pressure on hospital beds is necessitating a greater use of ambulatory treatment, is hard to say.

As Chapter 8 indicates, the trials comparing the outcomes of surgery and sclerotherapy in patients with varicose veins have tended to favour surgery as far as the incidence of late recurrences occur. Whether this matters very much is debatable; if late recurrences do occur, then one may argue reasonably that they can simply be re-injected. The inconvenience of this must be offset against the cost and the slight but real risk of general anaesthesia in those electing surgery. In addition, Fegan's technique – like other comparable techniques – is highly dependent on the skill, appropriateness and attention to detail with which it is applied. For this reason, it is to be expected that individual clinicians will get varying results from the technique, to a greater extent than might be the case with surgical treatment. This is not to denigrate the abilities of those who have advocated surgery, but rather to stress that clinicians committed to the technique may get better results than those who use it only occasionally.

A good example is Dr Labas of Bratislava, who presented his experience at the inaugural meeting of the European Venous Forum in June 2000. In a large series of 786 patients with venous ulceration, 82% completed a course of sclerotherapy using Fegan's method, with healing of the ulcer in 94.7% patients. The five-year recurrence rate was 25.7%, and all recurrent ulcers healed following further sclerotherapy. Randomised controlled trials are an effective way of conducting research, but excellent results such as these from personal series should be allowed to carry some weight.

What is the future for sclerotherapy? The development of foam sclerosants, as described by Cabrera of Granada, seems to many to be the most exciting development in the field. As Fegan has pointed out, it is likely that many of the poor results with sclerotherapy over the years have been due to injection into an inadequately emptied vein, resulting in simple thrombosis rather than fibrous obliteration. Foam sclerosant potentially overcomes this problem by displacing the blood within the vein, thus making the procedure easier to master. In addition, the foam is visible on ultrasound, allowing ultrasound-guided injections of, for example, the upper LSV to be performed accurately. Foam sclerotherapy of large venous malformations, with spectacular results, has been described recently by Cabrera.

In summary, what is the role of venous sclerotherapy? Most would agree that it is the treatment of choice for telangiectasia, and for minor recurrent or residual post-operative varicosities. Its place as a primary treatment for varicose veins with junctional incompetence is more controversial. Such controlled trials as have been done indicate a better long-term outcome after surgery. For many patients, however, the avoidance of general or spinal anaesthesia, the speed of treatment, and the absence of the need to take time off from work or looking after children will be important factors, leading to a steady demand for injection sclerotherapy. If Fegan's technique is followed meticulously, such patients can be reassured that they will be having an effective, safe, and (if necessary) easily repeatable treatment that is likely to give good results.

Further Reading

Abu-Own A, Scurr JH, Coleridge Smith PD (1993). Assessment of intermittent pneumatic compression by strain gauge plethysmography. *Phlebology* **8**:68–71.

Abu-Own A, Scurr JH, Coleridge Smith PD (1995). Effects of compression stockings on the skin microcirculation in chronic venous insufficiency. *Phlebology* **10**:5–11.

Abu-Own A, Shami SK, Chittenden SJ, Farrah J, Scurr JH, Coleridge Smith PD (1994). Microangiopathy of the skin and the effect of leg compression in patients with chronic venous insufficiency. *J Vasc Surg* **19**:1074–1083.

Adams EF (1849). *The Genuine Works of Hippocrates.* Sydenham Press, London.

Anning ST (1954). *Leg Ulcers – Their Causes and Treatment.* J&A Churchill Ltd., London.

Askar O, Abou-el-Ainen M (1963). The surgical anatomy of the deep fascia of the human leg (1). *J Cardiovasc Surg* **4**:114–125.

Baccaglini U, Spreafico G, Castoro C, Sorrentino P (1997). Consensus conference on sclerotherapy of varicose veins of the lower limb. *Phlebology* **12**:2–16.

Beresford SAA, Chant ADB, Jones HO, Piachaud D, Weddell JM (1978). Varicose veins: a comparison of surgery and injection/compression sclerotherapy – five year follow-up. *Lancet* **1**:921–924.

Braverman IM, Sibley J (1990). Ultrastructural and three-dimensional analysis of the contractile cells of the cutaneous microvasculature. *J Invest Dermatol* **95**:90–96.

Browse NL, Burnand KG, Lea Thomas M (1988). *Diseases of the Veins. Pathology, Diagnosis and Treatment.* Edward Arnold, London.

Champion RH (1970). Blood vessels and lymphatics of the skin. In Champion RH, Gillman T, Rook AJ, Sims RT (eds). *An Introduction to the Biology of the Skin.* Blackwell, Oxford.

Chant ADB, Jones HO, Weddell JM (1972). Varicose veins: a comparison of surgery and injection/compression sclerotherapy. *Lancet* **2**:1188–1191.

Cockett FB, Elgan-Jones DE (1953). The ankle blow-out syndrome. *Lancet* **1**:17–23.

Coleridge Smith PD (1990). Noninvasive venous investigation. *Vasc Med Rev* **1**:139–166.

Coleridge Smith PD, Scurr JH, Robinson KP (1987). Optimum methods of limb compression following varicose vein surgery. *Phlebology* **2**:165–172.

Dodd H, Cockett FB (1956). *The Pathology and Surgery of the Veins of the Lower Limb.* Livingstone, London.

Doran FSA, White M (1975). A clinical trial designed to discover if the primary treatment of varicose veins should be by Fegan's method or by an operation. *Br J Surg* **62**:72–76.

Einarsson E, Eklof B, Neglen P (1993). Sclerotherapy or surgery for varicose veins: a prospective randomized study. *Phlebology* **8**:22–26.

Fegan WG (1960). Continuous uninterrupted compression technique of injecting varicose veins. *Proc R Soc Med* **53**:837–.840

Fegan WG (1963). Continuous compression technique of injecting varicose veins. *Lancet* **ii**:109–112.

Galland RB, Magee TR, Lewis MH (1998). A survey of current attitudes of British and Irish vascular surgeons to venous sclerotherapy. *Eur J Vasc Endovasc Surg* **16**:43–46.

Gardner AMN, Fox RH (1983). The venous pump of the human foot. *Bristol Med Chir J* **98**:109–112.

Gardner AMN, Fox RH (1993). *The Return of Blood to the Heart*, 2nd edn. John Libby, London.

Gay J (1868). *On Varicose Disease of the Lower Extremity. The Lettsonian Lectures of 1867*. Churchill, London.

Hobbs JT (1974). Surgery and sclerotherapy in the treatment of varicose veins. *Arch Surg* 109:793-796.

Homans J (1917). The etiology and treatment of varicose ulcer of the leg. *Surg Gynecol Obstet* 24:300-311.

Jakobsen BH (1979). The value of different forms of treatment for varicose veins. *Br J Surg* 66:182-184.

Jones NAG, Webb PJ, Rees RI, Kakkar VV (1980). A physiological study of elastic compression stockings in venous disorders of the leg. *Br J Surg* 67:569-572.

Keller WL (1905). A new method of extirpating the internal saphenous and similar veins in varicose conditions. *New York Med J* 82:385-386.

Levick JR (1991). Capillary filtration-absorption balance reconsidered in the light of dynamic extravascular factors. *Exp Physiol* 76:825-857.

Linton RR (1938). The communicating veins of the lower leg and the operative technique for their ligation. *Ann Surg* 107:582-593.

Luscher TF (1991). Endothelium derived nitric oxide: the endogenous nitrovasodilator in the human cardiovascular system. *Eur Heart J* 12:2-11.

Mayberry JC, Moneta GL, De Frang RD, Porter JM (1991). The influence of elastic compression on deep venous haemodynamics. *J Vasc Surg* 13:91-99.

Mayo CH (1906). Treatment of varicose veins. *Surg Gynecol Obstet* 2:385-388.

Michel CC, Phillips ME (1987). Steady-state fluid filtration at different capillary pressures in perfused frog mesenteric capillaries. *J Physiol* 388:421-435.

Moretti G (1968). The blood vessels of the skin. In Gans 0, Steigleder GK (eds). *Jadassohn's Handbuch der Haut- und Geschlechtskrankheiten*, Vol. 1/1, pp. 491-623. Springer, Berlin.

Pegum JM, Fegan WG (1967). Anatomy of venous return from the foot. *Cardiovasc Res* 1:241-248.

Perrin M (1990). *L'Insuffisance Veineuse Chronique des Membres Inferieurs*. Medsi/McGraw-Hill, Paris.

Pfeifer JR, Hawtof GD (1989). Injection sclerotherapy and CO_2 laser sclerotherapy in the ablation of cutaneous spider veins of the lower extremity. *Phlebology* 4:231-240.

Reddy P, Wickers J, Terry T, Lamont P, Moller J, Dormandy JA (1986). What is the correct period of bandaging following sclerotherapy? *Phlebology* 1:217-220.

Rowden Foote R (1949). *Varicose Veins*. Butterworth, London.

Ruckley CV (1992). Treatment of venous ulceration: compression therapy. *Phlebology* 7 (**Suppl. 1**):22-26.

Ryan TJ (1970). Microvascular system and the skin. *Br J Hosp Med* 3:741-745.

Scott HJ (1990). Varicose veins and arteriovenous shunts – a review. *Phlebology* 5:77-83.

Seddon J (1973). The management of varicose veins. *Br J Surg* 60:345-347.

Sigg K (1952). The treatment of varicosities and accompanying complications. *Angiology* 355-379.

Smith FL, Johnson MA (1948). Incidence of pulmonary embolism after venous sclerosing therapy. *Minnesota Med J* 31:270.

Somerville JJF, Brow GO, Byrne PJ, Quill RD, Fegan WG (1974). The effect of elastic stockings on superficial venous pressures in patients with venous insufficiency. *Br J Surg* 61:979-981.

Spender JK (1868). *A Manual of the Pathology and Treatment of Ulcers and Subcutaneous Diseases of the Lower Limb*. Churchill, London.

Strandness DE Jr, Thiele BI (1981). *Selected Topics in Venous Disorders: Pathophysiology, Diagnosis and Treatment*. Futura, New York.

Trendelenburg F (1890). Uber die Unterbindung der Vena saphena magna bei Unterschenkelvaricen. *Bruns Beitr Klin Chir* 7:195-210.

Vanhoutte PM, Shepherd JT (1970) Effect of temperature on reactivity of isolated cutaneous veins of the dog. *Am J Physiol* 218:187-190.

Vanhoutte PM, Shepherd JT (1985). Adrenergic pharmacology of human and canine periph-
    eral veins. *Fed Proc* **44**:337–340.
Whitehead S, Lemenson G, Browse NL (1983). The assessment of calf pump function by iso-
    tope plethysmography. *Br J Surg* **70**:675–679.

Index